The Orgone Matrix

Unravelling the Mysteries of Orgonite

TERICA L. BRINK

ayana
crystals

ayana
crystals

ISBN-13: 9798372852860

Book and Cover design: Ralph N.

Printed in the United States of America

First Edition: January, 2023

CONTENTS

INTRODUCTION

O rgonite is the perfect emblem of the new-age. It is a mixing of the old and the new, combining the ancient earth magic of crystals and metal with the quantum leaps of our current era. Orgonite belongs to those who are ready to reach higher dimensions, to bring the flow of positive life energy back to a world where entropy seems unavoidable.

This book is more than just a how-to, it is a complete and comprehensive guide to making, using and understanding orgonite. It contains the answers to all of your questions about where orgonite comes from and how it works, as well as presenting unique perspectives from scientists and energy workers.

The Orgone Matrix is just another name for the energy-shifting layered metal and resin compound, but it also describes the complex context that it arose from. Orgonite doesn't exist in a void, it is part of a bigger theory, part of a lifestyle that is centered on upliftment, progress and the wellbeing of individuals, societies and the world itself. The theory is based on the idea that a fundamental force of nature has been overlooked by many of the institutions that govern the functioning of society.

If you are curious about orgonite, this book will guide you through the history, art and science of the orgone matrix. Each section features a blend of technique and narrative to bring you a comprehensive understanding of how this concept is being used as well as the philosophy and science from which it emerged. There is a fine line between mystery and misinformation; the impartial observations presented here will give you the confidence to navigate the tumult of information out there, formulate your own opinions and apply the knowledge in a useful way. In addition to the instructional elements, you will come to understand the community that orgonite represents: people who believe that there is something more to life, that there are alternative ways of doing things and that those options are worthy of exploration and development. Although entire books have been written on that topic alone, a few sections of this book shine a light on how the flow of information is controlled and the risk independent thinkers have faced when operating outside of the mainstream.

Orgonite simply represents one of the many ways of accessing or interacting with the innate resonant energy of our universe and introduces a new lexicon, a new framework for understanding the potentials of improving our relationship with this resource in all areas of our lives.

The information in The Orgone Matrix has been arranged into four main parts which do not necessarily need to be read in a linear fashion - you are welcome to jump into the section that catches your interest first. Part 1 discusses orgonite and its origins, while Part 2 is a practical guide to making it at home. Part 3 explains the various scientific and philosophical concepts associated with orgonite and the last section takes a closer look at the life of Wilhelm Reich, the scientist that gave Orgone its name and the controversy he caused with his ideas and inventions. Each topic can be explored in much greater detail in books and online, so the bibliography also functions as a list of recommendations for further reading and exploration.

PART - I

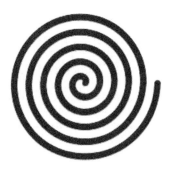

Understanding The Orgone Matrix

CHAPTER ONE

WHAT ON EARTH IS ORGONITE?

T he idea of the ether has been prevalent throughout human history, since science and mysticism were intertwined. Many people believe in the subtle field or force of life-giving energy, if only as an abstract medium in which the other proven forces of nature manifest and interact. Even Einstein, whose theory of special relativity negated the Newtonian concept of ether, agreed that the "empty" space between objects has its own properties. The idea has been debated for as long as it has existed and has been called by many different names, although the concepts remain similar.

Some of the names you might have heard are prana, which comes from Vedic tradition, or Qi, from the Buddhists. On the other side of the planet, words like odyle, elan vital and Orgone have been used. There is seemingly endless information available about subjective experiences with this subtle life force energy, yet it is ultimately considered unscientific, or pseudoscientific, as there is very little objective research available and almost nothing that verifies its existence by the parameters of classical physics. Rather, there is a distinct implication in the mainstream science community that to try to investigate such a concept is not only a waste of time, but also somewhat embarrassing.

Although the various names all refer to essentially the same thing, Orgone stands out as this was the name given to that fundamental energy by a psychoanalyst-turned-scientist who worked tirelessly to quantize its properties and effects using the methods of classical science and biology of his time. For his efforts, he had bestowed upon him the honor of two book burnings on two different continents, a federal injunction that prevented him from distributing his books and devices, and a prison sentence that ended with his untimely death in 1957, just days before a parole hearing. That scientist was Wilhelm Reich, a controversial figure who has not faded into obscurity the way that those who were against him might have hoped. In fact, decades of lingering interest in his discoveries and new inventions based on his ideas are what led to the publication of this book.

In the new age of spirituality and openness to the idea that there is vital energy that permeates the universe, many people are looking for ways to interact with this energy and understand its effects on our bodies, minds and environments. Physical practices like yoga, tai chi and reiki are growing in popularity, as well as less obvious techniques like sound and crystal healing. However, these practices are geared more towards influencing the individual than the environment. In the early 1990s, based on Reich's theories of Orgone, a product was invented that claims to passively accumulate and concentrate this ethereal energy, which can have immense positive effects on environmental as well as personal wellbeing.

The product is a mixture of metal and quartz, cast in resin, which forms a matrix that attracts life-positive energy, thereby diminishing the effects of entropy and decay. The self-proclaimed original inventor, Karl Hans Welz, chose to call it Orgonite™, based on Reich's name for the ubiquitous energy, however he did not trademark the name until much later, by which time others had latched on to the name, using it as a generic term to describe their own versions of the substance.

There are a lot of claims about what the orgone-matrix can do, but very little explanation as to how it works or where it came from. In an effort to answer those questions, this book takes a deep dive back to the beginning of the 20th century, to discover how we got from Orgone to orgonite.

The main claims about orgonite are that it balances harmful or negative energy and promotes positive and healing energy. It gets used in gardens, homes and a large community of people "gift" orgonite to the environment. Anecdotal evidence suggests that orgonite can improve quality of sleep, facilitate better health and a stronger sense of well-being. Gardeners have noted an improvement in growth by simply burying a piece of orgonite among their plants and people that are considered to be hypersensitive to electromagnetic fields use the product to diminish the effects that they experience due to the constant exposure to man-made radiation that is a seemingly unavoidable part of modern life.

It is used to make plates that "charge up" food and water, in a similar way to the experiments done by Dr. Maseru Emoto that show how the crystalline structure of water changes in response to different energies and intentions. For personal protection, it can be worn as a pendant or carried in a pocket. Certain corners of the Internet overflow with documentation of at-home experimentation that shows off all of these marvelous effects, yet very few can explain exactly how they are achieved by these seemingly inert little polymer artefacts. Even within the orgonite community, such as it is, there are different factions who often disagree on the techniques of making and using orgonite, as well as the reliability of the scientific reasoning behind their effectiveness.

At first glance, understanding orgonite seems simple, as there is an abundance of websites that confidently assert the ways that it can change your life by sucking up all the bad vibes and turning them into good ones. Unsurprisingly, nearly all of these sites promote their own orgone matrix products and unfailingly suggest that the more pieces of orgonite you have, the more benefits you will receive.

There have also been many attempts at describing the science behind it all, yet very few of the people producing orgone-matrix materials have read any of Reich's original research and so they often overlook some of the most fundamental aspects of working with orgone energy. Instead, they rely on poorly understood concepts pilfered from the world of electrophysics to offer explanations that are impenetrable to the layman, yet patently false to material scientists.

Reich himself tried for years to reconcile his work with the classical model of physics, but to no avail, so pretending that the two systems are fully compatible ultimately discredits Reich's model which is perfectly consistent within itself and is the sole reason for orgonite's existence in the first place. Orgonite doesn't resemble anything that Wilhelm Reich would have had in his laboratory in his day, but his research forms the foundation of the principles that are used in the making of it in the present.

CHAPTER TWO

MORE THAN ROCKS AND GLITTER

O rgonite is primarily found in online stores, at craft fairs or in those weird and wonderful boutiques that sell all sorts of spiritual esoterica, from crystals and tarot cards to pendulums and singing bowls. The pieces come in a variety of shapes, colors and designs and can include a variety of elements like whole crystals, copper coils or similar conductive materials, and symbolic tokens. Some orgone-matrix pieces have visible layers set in transparent resin that allows you to see all the elements contained within, whereas others are opaque with a more uniform distribution of materials. Depending on where you're getting your information from, some of these pieces are unfortunately nothing more than objets d'art, far more effective at weighting down papers than creating the energy-cleansing vortices that they are supposed to.

Google trends data reveals that searches for "orgonite" are on the rise, while searches for "orgone" have decreased since 2004 which suggests that more people are interested in orgonite itself than the science behind it. Because of this, the true technique of making it has been abandoned in favor of designs that appeal to the aesthetic sensibilities. That is not to say that every beautiful orgonite piece is fake or intended to dupe the buyer for the sake of a quick profit, it is just that the science of Orgone (Orgonomy) has been neglected, or perhaps simply misinterpreted by those who seek to promote this crystalline cure-all.

Of course, as awareness of orgone matrix devices and their potential effects has increased, more people have added their personal ideas and interpretations to its development. As you can see in the image, there are several distinct styles which are representative of the different schools of thought surrounding the product. To the uninitiated, it is very difficult to determine which is "real" orgonite, so let's examine each style individually to clarify where they came from and the ideas that inspired them.

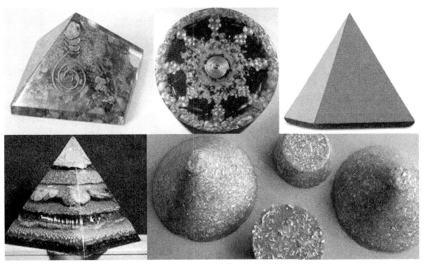

Karl H Welz: Orgonite™

This is the dark gray opaque pyramid in the top right image. In his autobiographical notes, Karl Welz describes himself as a life-long student of the esoteric arts, so he was already familiar with the concept of an underlying life force energy via his interactions with prana and chi when he encountered the work of his fellow Austrian, Wilhelm Reich. One of the most important devices Reich invented was the Orgone Accumulator, which did exactly what the name suggests. The device was a box that was made by layering organic and inorganic materials, such as wood or plastic and metal, which would concentrate Orgone energy inside the box. The more layers of material, the more effective the device would be.

Welz contrived to condense as many layers as possible in a much smaller format, which is how he came to the idea of embedding minuscule particles of iron (inorganic material) within a carbon-based resin (organic) to create the first metal-resin matrix intended for energy accumulation. He has since added quartz powder into his formula and over the years, his technique has been refined and modified to work in conjunction with the Orgone-generating Radionics devices that are his primary interest, although he insists that the pyramids and pendants, he produces are effective on their own as well. No one can really claim to own the concept of Orgone accumulation, since even Reich himself was not the first to conceive of it, but the first person to bring the word "orgonite" into the world was definitely Karl Hans Welz. He currently owns the trademark on the name and his specific recipe, although he has been met with complaints for trying to enforce the trademark on what many consider a generic term.

Don Croft: Orgone Pyramids, HHGs, Towerbusters and more…

On the bottom right you can see the silvery cones and discs with visible metal particles. Like Welz, Don Croft was interested in building Orgone Accumulators and frequency-generating healing devices (he called his a "Zapper"). He admits that he took inspiration from Welz's technique for his own designs, but he believed that he had improved them under the guidance of his psychic and energy-sensitive wife and daughter. The metal particles in Croft's orgone matrix formula are much larger and every piece includes one or more whole crystals, preferably double-terminated and often wrapped with a mobius coil. Croft relied much more on the subtle energy effects his energy-perceptive family could see taking place than the original Orgonomic science and subsequently came up with a variety of products with unique ingredients, shapes and forms that were designed to affect the environment in different ways.

Don and his wife Carol believed that their orgonite was superior because the addition of crystals and conductive coils made the products capable of neutralizing negative energy as well as enhancing positive energy. They were responsible for pioneering the culture of "gifting" - strategically placing orgonite around areas of negative energy - and have chronicled their gifting adventures all over the United States and the world. This type of orgonite is most prevalent online and there are hundreds of resources explaining how to make and use the different forms.

The other pieces you can see are the more recent artistic interpretations of the Croft-style orgonite, derisively called "glitterite" by those who think they are better informed. These are obviously intended for display, whereas both the Welz and the original Croft designs prioritize function over aesthetics. The function, however, has been a matter of intense debate among the two groups, who can't quite agree on how orgonite actually works. To get to the root of this issue and form your own opinion about whose technique is more viable, it is important to understand some of the concepts, terminology and instruments that come from the original field of Orgone research.

CHAPTER THREE

THE FUNDAMENTALS OF ORGONE

"The energy was named "orgone," in reference to the history of its discovery through the study of the orgasm and to its biological effect of charging substances of organic origin. Now I was able to understand the blue-gray vapors that I had seen in the dark around my head, hands, and white coat: organic matter absorbs Orgone energy and retains it." - Wilhelm Reich, The Cancer Biopathy

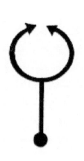

R eich used this symbol to describe how Orgone energy is the connecting point that underpins both mechanistic and mystical worldviews. His initial work in psychoanalysis and medicine enabled him to understand that physical and non-physical phenomena are simply two aspects of one reality, not only in terms of the individual mind-body matrix but at a universal level. He concluded that Orgone energy was the underlying force of atmospheric and cosmic processes, consciousness and life itself, meaning movement, biogenesis, reproduction, growth and even evolution. It is clearly stated that it is neither electromagnetic nor material in nature, but rather the medium in which these phenomena appear and interact.

The particular properties of Orgone that Reich declared after years of observation are as follows:

- It is mass free.
- It is omnipresent.
- It is the medium in which electromagnetic and gravitational phenomena take place.
- It is in constant motion.
- It is antithetical to entropy (some people use the word negentropic).
- It forms units of creative energy, meaning living or non-living units that acquire energy from the environment.
- It creates matter.
- It generates life.
- It is self-attracted and capable of superimposition.
- It can be manipulated with the appropriate devices.

Since Reich's own body of work consists of more than twenty manuscripts and publications, not to mention the affirming work that has been done in the years following his death, it would be tedious to discuss all of the research and evidence that lead to these claims, however a list of recommended texts is appended for those who are curious.

Reich first became interested in the idea of a biophysical energy after studying Freud's theory of Libido under the guidance of Freud himself. In his early experiments he became aware that sexual excitation could be measured as a directly proportional electrical charge on the skin. His speculations on the nature of this energy were explored in his first major publication, The Function of the Orgasm, which would later be revised and republished as the first volume of The Discovery of Orgone, once he had come to understand how this original work had informed his later revelations. One of the key observations he made at this point of his research was the idea that energy manifesting measurably in the body displays the properties of expansion and contraction. He went on to integrate this knowledge with his psychoanalytic theory of Character Analysis to create a psycho-physical therapeutic practice called Vegetotherapy.

Volume II of The Discovery of Orgone was a book that was originally titled *The Cancer Biopathy* and featured some of the most important of his investigative ventures: *The Bion Experiments*. These revealed that bacteriological life forms could emerge from sterile and inanimate solutions under certain conditions, in the form of blue-glowing vesicles that Reich called *Bions*. From these experiments, Reich began to elaborate on his observation that there was a unique force governing the interactions between energy and matter. In nearly all of his experiments, Reich would describe the soft blue glow that indicated a strong saturation of Orgone energy, appearing like an aura around the object of his study. An organism's health could be determined by the state of this blue glowing aura, which is notably diminished in damaged or decaying cells. There is photographic documentation that suggests Reich was even able to record the presence of Orgone in a vacuum, which has been repeated by contemporary Orgone researcher, James DeMeo.

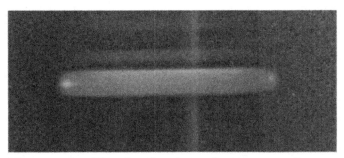

Figure 6: Blue lumination of ~450 nm, from a high-vacuum (0.5 micron) pressure glass tube, charged in a strong orgone accumulator over a year. No electricity was applied. The tube glows only from hand-stroking. (DeMeo 2002a)

The famous invention, of course, is the Orgone Accumulator. The study of expansion and contraction of this biological energy led Reich to seek ways of facilitating expansion and amplification of the primordial force. Through his work, Reich had noticed that organic materials and water seemed to attract Orgone, whereas inorganic metals would deflect or repel it. From this, the idea of layering the two different materials evolved, which had the measurable effect of creating a higher charge on the inside of a box that had been manufactured in this fashion. This higher charge of etheric energy could be imparted to whichever person or thing happened to be inside of the box, allowing them to draw directly on the life force itself, although some people did report adverse effects of overexposure, such as hot flushes, skin tingling and increased pulse.

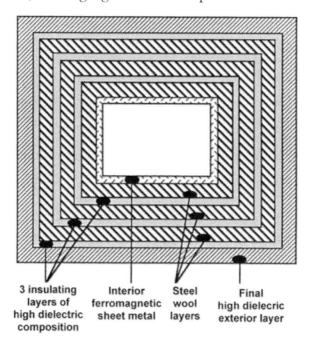

3 insulating layers of high dielectric composition   Interior ferromagnetic sheet metal   Steel wool layers   Final high dielecric exterior layer

Inside an Orgone Accumulator

Another critical experiment that forever changed the way Reich viewed his own breakthrough was the ORANUR Experiment, or Experiment XX, which proved that concentrated Orgone works, metaphorically, like an electric current: it doesn't matter what you plug in, it will switch on. This effect has many benefits, of course, but can be detrimental too, as an Orgone Accumulator does not discriminate between "good" and "bad" energetic phenomena.

A plant placed inside an Orgone Accumulator (ORAC) will flourish thanks to the abundance of vital energy; a milligram of radioactive material placed inside an ORAC will immediately poison everyone in the laboratory and increase the background radiation level throughout a 600 mile radius. The disastrous experiment, which actually took place in New England, was brought to a halt when he realized that the radiation effects did not diminish even after the radioactive material was removed from the property. The increased background radiation levels were even reported in the news on February 3rd 1951, although it was officially attributed to atomic bomb experiments taking place in the desert halfway across the country.

What Reich had inadvertently discovered in this experiment was that Orgone energy is agitated by certain types of radiation and electromagnetic activity. Exposure to these particular radio-frequencies disrupts the structure and behavior of Orgone and creates instability in the affected environment. Further observation revealed the excessively excited Orgone did not return to its original state, but rather persisted in this volatile condition until it became "burnt out" and took on a deadened, immobile character which Reich called DOR - Deadly Orgone Radiation. From that point forward, Reich would refer to Orgone in its natural, negentropic state as POR (Positive Orgone Radiation) in contrast to the corrupted, hyper-entropic state known as Oranur (Orgone Against Nuclear Radiation) and the stagnant DOR.

In POR and DOR, Reich saw a further embodiment of his initial theories about the expanding and contracting nature of bioenergy, with POR representing the ripe and blooming expansive counterpart to the shrivelled and tightening contractions of DOR.

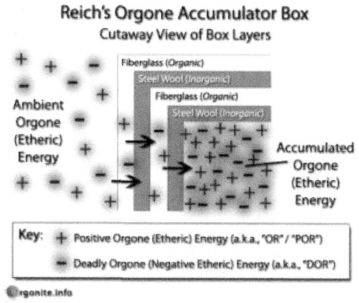

A visualization of orgone energy passing through the layers of an orgone accumulator.

Once he was satisfied that Orgone and its effects were real and measurable, Reich started to test the application of the Orgone Accumulator in improving people's health. He understood that not every condition would benefit from exposure to concentrated Orgone, particularly hypertensive conditions where a more excited cellular state is likely to do more harm than good. After the ORANUR Experiments, Reich also became aware that environmental conditions would be hugely important in administering Orgone-based therapy and stipulated that his devices should not be used within range of broadcasting towers and receivers, energy production plants, especially nuclear, and even fluorescent light bulbs should be avoided.

The best place to use an Orgone accumulating device would be in an open, natural environment where the risk of creating or amplifying negative or "deadly" Orgone is drastically reduced, and so it became common for Orgone Accumulators to be built and used outside in rural areas.

In response to his observations of Oranur and DOR, Reich concluded that modern technology was contributing to the increasing instability of the environment, particularly in regard to a phenomenon known as desertification. Because Orgone has a direct influence on atmospheric processes like weather patterns and cloud formation, it followed that these natural processes could be experiencing disruptions due to advancements in nuclear technology and the proliferation of areas affected by man-made electromagnetic fields and radiation. He had also observed that exposure to DOR resulted in a type of sickness affecting the human body in a similar way to the environment, particularly by stagnating the natural processes and allowing a deadening or dullness to occur; a desertification of the spirit.

In an attempt to counteract these negative effects, Reich invented another device which he called a Cloudbuster. Using the knowledge he had learned about the behavior of Orgone, particularly its properties of attraction and superimposition, he would target areas where Orgone appeared to be stagnant or where DOR had built up, to encourage the return to a healthy flow of positive Orgone. The Cloudbuster consisted of an array of metal pipes connected to a flowing body of water, which would be pointed at the sky to first attract and then "drain off" the stagnant or entropic energy, so that the free flow of Orgone could resume and restore the harmonious balance of the environment.

The Cloudbuster had its own set of complicated rules for engagement to avoid causing further damage, so its use was restricted to only his most experienced and trusted colleagues in a project he called CORE - Cosmic Orgone Engineering. After several decades of trying to understand the life force energy on earth, Reich broadened his horizons to consider the extra-terrestrial implications of living on a planet that seemed to possess its own innate qualities of Orgone accumulation. Reich even predicted that Earth would be enveloped in a blue-glowing atmosphere, which wouldn't be confirmed until the first satellite photos of the planet were transmitted two years after his death. In his final book, Contact with Space, Reich expresses his belief that his cosmic engineering had led him to encounters with agents that were using advanced Orgone technology to power air or space crafts and aspired to build his own motor devices that could draw on this abundant natural energy.

For Reich, Orgone had the potential to become a Grand Unified Theory on a philosophical and scientific scale. Given the proper attention, he presumed Orgonomy in all its facets might offer the solution to all of humanity's ills by harnessing the power of Orgone to cure medical and psychological ailments and provide mechanisms and infrastructure to end pollution, resource scarcity and the harsh divide of inequality that he considered a plague on societal health.

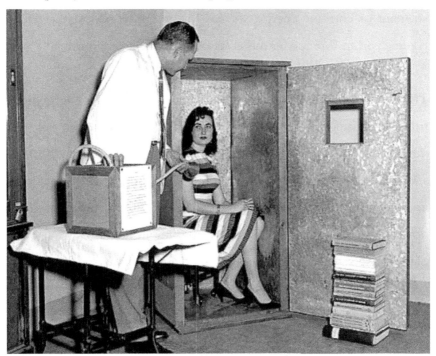

A patient inside the ORAC

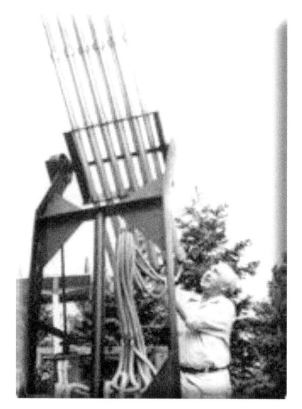

Cosmic Engineering with the Cloudbuster

CHAPTER FOUR

FROM ORGONE TO ORGONITE: A PRIMORDIAL ENERGY'S JOURNEY

For various reasons which are discussed in more detail in the chapter about Reich and the conspiracy against him, the FDA decided he was a fraud, and banned his devices and most of his books, which they considered to be "promotional literature". When the injunction that forbade the transport of ORACs across state lines was accidentally breached by a colleague who was transferring an ORAC to a storage unit, both Reich and the colleague, Dr. Silvert were sent to prison. Reich accurately and tragically predicted that he would not survive his two-year sentence and Dr. Silvert took his own life within a year of his release, so it is no wonder that many still view this case with a degree of suspicion. Reich had known there would be no acceptance of his theories in his lifetime and had instructed that his collection of original research remain sealed until 50 years after his death, in order to protect his ideas until a more enlightened and unbiased world could investigate them fairly. This, combined with the ban on his books about Orgone, could explain why so many false narratives about Reich and his discoveries persisted in the years following his death.

The Orgone Accumulator and its persecuted inventor had acquired a bit of a cult status among the counterculture movements of the 1960s, thanks to their interest in free energy and free love, and by the 1970s a very small group of people were still interested in the weather-engineering prospects of the Cloudbuster, most notably James DeMeo, who is still actively involved in Orgone research today. Reich's two major inventions enjoyed some prevalence in alternative communities right up until the 1980s when both Welz and Croft started to build and experiment with Orgone Accumulators for themselves.

Among the first variations of the Orgone Accumulator that Reich developed were the wand and funnel, which would be used to direct the condensed orgone energy from inside an accumulator box. This would be used for acute treatment of physical ailments to accelerate the healing process. An orgone blanket works in a similar way, and was designed for those who were too unwell to visit a therapist with an orgone accumulator. Using the same principle of layering, the blanket was made of steel wool encased in fabric, so that it could be wrapped around the patient. Smaller versions were also used for treatment of specific parts of the body, like a wounded limb for example.

After the discovery of DOR came the Cloudbuster, with its long metal pipes and the ability to change the weather. The success with this device encouraged Reich to develop a tiny version, the medical DOR-buster which was a hand-held instrument that worked according to the same principle of draining off negative energy. These were the only tools that were used in the ongoing study of Reich's work until the invention of Orgonite™ in 1992, which spawned an entire new generation of orgone devices, like the Chembusters, Terminators and Generators. What's interesting, however, is this charming story told by Don Croft, which proves that the orgone-matrix has no known inventor and relies on a concept that existed long before patents and trademarks:

"Stacie sat on the beach at Cape Hatteras' Outer Bank last weekend and baited hooks for a knowledgeable old black gentleman who had made his own fishing weights of fiberglass resin, BBs (small ball bearings) and a quartz crystal. His grandfather taught him to do that and he apparently catches more fish than anyone around."Stacie sat on the beach at Cape Hatteras' Outer Bank last weekend and baited hooks for a knowledgeable old black gentleman who had made his own fishing weights of fiberglass resin, BBs (small ball bearings) and a quartz crystal. His grandfather taught him to do that and he apparently catches more fish than anyone around.

'Granpappy was poor... loved to fish. And couldn't afford weights but could always get hold of old cans [cut into little bits] and pine sap and energy rocks.'

The fisherman calls his sinkers 'energy stones' so if anyone asks who invented orgonite, the short answer is that nobody alive can claim credit for it."

When Welz created his Orgone Generator in 1991, he believed that he had created something far more powerful than the original Orgone Accumulator, something that could eliminate negative DOR energy while amplifying the positive life energy. Orgonite™ was invented as a component of this electronically powered device. The idea behind the metal-resin matrix is that it allows the same process that takes place via the multiple layers of an ORAC to happen at an exponentially higher rate due to the thousands upon thousands of layers that are formed by the suspension of inorganic metal particles in the organic polymer. In this way, a piece of Orgonite™ is said to act as a magnet for life force energy, which then absorbs and stores it, almost like a battery. Although the exact design of the Orgone Generator is confidential, the theory seems to be that running a charge through Orgonite™ will create a continuous flow of pulsating Positive Orgone energy that is capable of disrupting and restructuring any stagnant

DOR in the environment. The company that currently handles the production and distribution of Welz's products unequivocally states that Orgonite™ alone cannot generate or restructure energy, only attract it, and for that reason precautions should be taken to avoid amplifying DOR or negative frequencies.

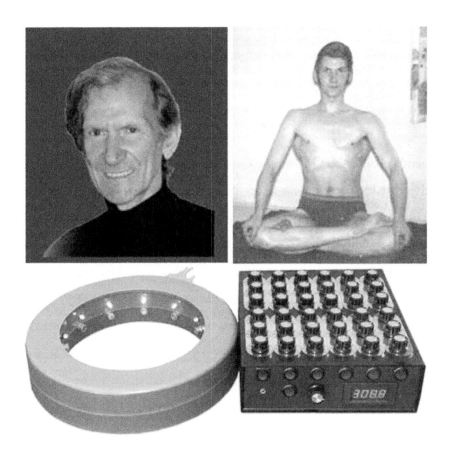

Karl H Welz and his Orgone Generator

Since the patent is still active on Welz's Orgonite™, specific recipes are not given and his videos seem to be provided to inspire personal experimentation rather than make exact replicas, but the basic formula is a 50-50 mixture of iron powder and epoxy. In a 2009 video he mentions "super" Orgonite™, but doesn't reveal the classified ingredient. However, a much more recent website lists quartz powder when describing the products, citing its association with having the quality of amplifying positive energy, rather than the piezoelectric effect which is often erroneously referred to. There is more information about this and other electromagnetic and quantum effects in the third section of this book. It's probably safe to assume that quartz is the classified ingredient that was hinted at over a decade before and the updated website also clarifies the use of iron being due to its resonance with the human body and blood. A colleague working closely with Welz and his son implies that any metal can be used, as it is the particle size that dictates the strength of the piece rather than the metal itself. Various metals each have their own qualities and resonance, so it is ultimately a matter of personal preference.

Having examined one of Welz's generators, Croft started to play around with his version of the Orgone matrix material, feeling much stronger energetic effects from crystals when used together with the metallic polymer compound. He too incorporated it into an electronic device called a Terminator, a small electrode plated machine that emitted specific frequencies that were supposed to help rid the body of disease-causing bacteria and parasites. His partner, Carol, alleged that the human aura responded fantastically to the presence of the orgonite-enhanced Terminator and they started experimenting with adding crystals into the formula in order to incorporate their healing effects.

Crystals are believed to have their own innate energetic qualities as well as the property of being programmable, meaning they can store a "memory" of a specific frequency. The Crofts charged their crystals with the waveform generated by the Terminator before wrapping them in highly conductive mobius coils and setting them within a metal-resin matrix, concluding that this would allow the final product to passively project a strong field of POR and transmute any DOR in the environment. In his personal records, Don suggests that this formula had the potential to neutralize radioactivity and so they began making vast quantities of orgonite to place around areas that were perceived to be concentrated with DOR. The popular name "Towerbuster" originated, in reference to the thick, hockey-puck style orgonite pieces intended to eliminate the negative energy produced by broadcasting towers.

The Crofts' claim that their inclusion of charged crystals made the pieces so powerful that it was not necessary to use expensive metal powder to create the magnified accumulation effect, but instead any metal shavings of any size could be used. The crystals would be different depending on the particular device, but they generally preferred double-terminated quartz which would be charged and placed in a specific arrangement according to the shape of the mold. Using the same theory of energy polarization (transmuting POR to DOR), they went on to create a modified and much smaller version of the Cloudbuster, choosing to set copper pipes into an orgone matrix rather than having to connect them to a body of water or Orgone Accumulator to draw off the toxic energy. This device was called a Chembuster as it was primarily used for dissolving Chemtrails in the same way that Reich and his cosmic engineers had dissolved stagnant DOR clouds. Croft admits that his device was not as effective as the original, though he considered it far safer due to its passive polarizing effect which allowed them to avoid the issue of exposure to concentrated DOR which had been a major downside of the original design. Work with the Chembuster is typically centered on cloud dissolution, with an abundance of images submitted to online forums showing the characteristic "blue hole" that appears in a cloud bank in direct alignment with the positioning of the Chembuster.

Don and Carol had become somewhat famous in the new-age and alternative communities because of their activism, encouraging as many people as possible to start buying or making their own orgonite and "gifting" it wherever it was deemed necessary to help rid the world of toxic radiation and negative energy. Although Don Croft lost his life in an unfortunate accident in 2018, prolific gifting movements are still active, one of the most prominent being Orgonize Africa, run by one of his longtime followers, Georg Ritschl. Some people were and still are very skeptical of the Crofts' claims, suggesting that their products are at best ineffective and at worst extremely harmful. Welz does not accept that a charged crystal provides enough energy to restructure corrupted Orgone and points out the imprudence of placing potential amplifiers in a radioactive environment. In turn, the Crofts accused Karl Welz of being overly attached to his status as the inventor of Orgonite™, noting that his devices produce "less blue and violet orgone" and the inclusion of powdered quartz produces a "hot, chaotic energy." Each of them addressed this contention on their websites and message boards where they remain for curious minds to peruse at their own leisure.

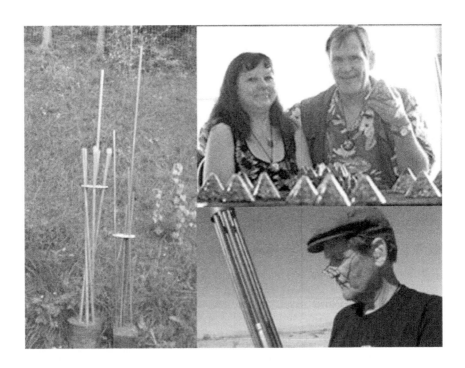

PART - II

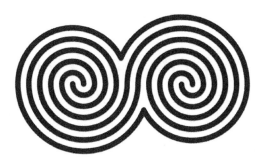

Making Orgone Matrix Models

CHAPTER FIVE

DIY ORGONITE

I f you would like to make your own orgone matrix, it is worth exploring the different forums and communities to see what resonates with you, as opinion on what is and is not effective is fairly polarized. You could even try both methods and see for yourself. The key beliefs of each faction are important, for instance, followers of Croft's technique are unambiguous in their suggestion that the power of a coil-wrapped, energetically charged crystal embedded in a metal-resin matrix will eliminate DOR from the atmosphere, generate positive energy and should be used to neutralize any unwanted electro-magnetic energy. Their development of orgone matrix products is based heavily on perception of psychic phenomena and does not draw on the original science of Orgonomy in the same way as Welz, but this has had little impact on the size of the community still actively using their methods and claiming to achieve remarkable results.

The team that works with Welz do not believe that the piezoelectric effect can take place within the crystalline orgone matrix, nor do they advise tactical gifting. In the other devices that Welz invented, namely Chi or Orgone Generators™, Welz relies on an external electrical charge to activate the Orgone generating components via a complex and confidential circuitry which can then be used in combination with Radionics technology to adjust the frequency of the energy. The producers claim that a Structural Link can be created between the Orgone Generator and the Orgonite™ Pyramid or pendant that allows it to work towards a specific intention at any distance. According to the website, it is not necessary to have a Generator for your Orgonite™ piece to be effective, but it is important to note that Orgonite™ itself does not generate Orgone energy, it simply attracts and amplifies what is already available.

Before learning where to place your orgonite, consider some of the claims that are being made about how it interacts with radiofrequency, or EMF. If you feel there is not enough evidence supporting the "restructuring" qualities of orgonite, why indeed would you choose to throw a chunk of the stuff directly under a cell tower? If Reich's Oranur Experiments teach us anything, it is to be extremely careful when using Orgone accumulating devices in the presence of harmful radiation. Although the radiation emitted by electromagnetic technology, such as radio and cell towers is considered "harmless" because of its non-ionizing nature, even the WHO admits that there is not enough information to accurately make that assumption and classifies all man-made radiofrequency emissions as "potentially carcinogenic." This goes for personal electronics too - sticking a piece of orgonite on your wi-fi router or on the back of your phone could turn out to be quite the mistake if the orgone matrix is not restructuring the DOR.

Like Welz combines his Orgone technology with Radionics, there are many other technologies that orgonite can work in tandem with, especially when it comes to frequency and resonance. The structure of crystals is said to provide them with their own "intelligence" which acts like a memory and allows them to carry certain programming. Since it's possible to imbue your crystals with a particular resonance which they will hold onto, many producers of orgonite today are using charged or programmed crystals in their devices in a similar way to Croft's use of his Terminator or "Zapper". At the end of this section is a list of popular resonances and frequencies to work with.

If you would prefer to err on the side of caution, apply the same limitations Reich laid out for his original accumulators: that is, keep the devices away from synthetic EMFs and use them rather where positively structured Orgone can already be found. Orgone attracts

Orgone, so this method will work to build up a strong field of positive energy and eliminate DOR naturally without running the risk of accidentally accumulating toxic energy. One of the ways the earth naturally restructures DOR is through grounding – which is why Reich used a run-off when working with Cloudbusters. One of the safest ways you can use orgonite is to plant it in your garden where it can boost your plant growth and won't pick up any DOR. Once your garden is flourishing, even more Orgone will be attracted to your environment and intensified. Reich noted that out of all the elements, Orgone has the strongest affinity with water and so it is often suggested to place orgonite pieces in or near a running stream or a water feature. The free-moving energy is already generating positive Orgone, so it serves as an optimal environment to use the orgonite.

Preparation

Here is a list of everything you will need to make your own orgone matrix material:

- epoxy resin and hardener
- metal powder (iron, copper, etc)
- measuring jug
- mixing stick
- protective gear - gloves, mask, eyewear
- molds
- vegetable oil
- crystals, coils or quartz powder (optional)

Working with a chemical product like epoxy resin can be intimidating, but following some simple rules will help. Epoxy does have a very strong smell and emits fumes that can be damaging to the lungs, so it is recommended that you work in a well-ventilated area with a high-quality mask covering your nose and mouth. Some people prefer to wear goggles or safety glasses to prevent eye sensitivity. Latex or rubber gloves will also be useful as the chemicals can cause an allergic reaction, and even if it doesn't, sticky resin on the skin is unpleasant and difficult to remove.

Resin is available in high-viscosity and low-viscosity variants, which refers to the thickness of the liquid. The different variants are designed for different applications, so there will be a difference in curing times and techniques that you can use. For the purposes of creating orgonite, low viscosity resin is suitable as it sets within 12-24 hours, deeper layers can be poured and it is easier to prevent air bubbles from getting trapped.

Epoxy resin normally comes in two liquid parts, the resin and a hardener, or catalyst, which reacts with the resin to allow it to form a solid, high-gloss plastic. Different brands may have different ratios for mixing the resin and hardener, so make sure you check the product you are using. Once the catalyst has been mixed in, you normally get about 45 minutes of working time before the resin starts to set. You will notice the consistency become thicker the longer you leave it, so it is best to set up your molds and materials before preparing the epoxy.

Remember, the layers you see in decorative orgonite pieces do not contribute to its effect, it is the matrix of layers created by the suspension of metal particles in resin that attracts Orgone energy, but if you would like your pieces to be more artistic, feel free to work layer by later, allowing hardening time between each pour.

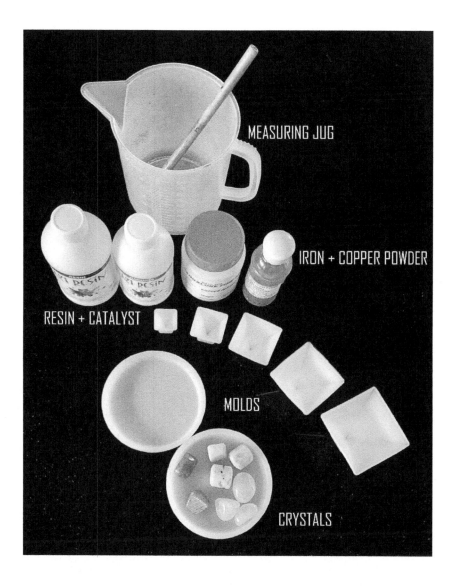

Step-by-step Instructions

- Fill each of the molds that you plan to use with water, then empty them all into the measuring jug and take note of the measurement. This is so you know how much epoxy mixture to pour. Empty and dry the jug.

- Dry the molds thoroughly, then brush on a thin layer of oil to make it easier to remove the product one it has set. If you are using silicon molds, oil may not be necessary.

- Check the ratio of resin to hardener recommended by the manufacturer, then calculate how much of each you need to pour, using the volume of water you recorded as a reference. Account for displacement if you are planning on using large crystals.

- Mix the resin and hardener together, then add approximately 2 teaspoons of metal powder per 100ml.

- (Optional) Add 1tsp of quartz powder per 100ml

- Pour the mixture into the molds, leaving enough space to add in whole crystals/other elements.

- Gently tap or shake the molds to release any air bubbles

- Make sure your molds are on a level surface and safe from any disturbances while you leave them to set. Depending on the climate this can take anywhere from a couple of hours to 24 hours.

- Carefully remove your orgone matrix piece from the mold and check for imperfections. Any untidy edges or flaws can be buffed away with sand paper.

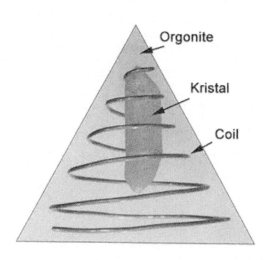

Above is a simple example of how conducting elements can be added to the orgone matrix, but it is important to know that the art of making these forms is subjective and personal. It is highly recommended that you use your own intuition to make devices that resonate with you and for you; through experience you will understand what works best. Once you have mastered the simple recipe above, explore some different techniques and materials using the tables on the following pages.

Multi-layer Designs:

If you want to see distinct layers of different materials or elements, it is important to allow the resin to set firmly in between each session of pouring. Remember that the number of visible layers does not affect the piece's potency, however it does make for an appealing design. To reveal the crystal or other elements within, pour a thin, clear layer of resin around the element when you set it in the mold.

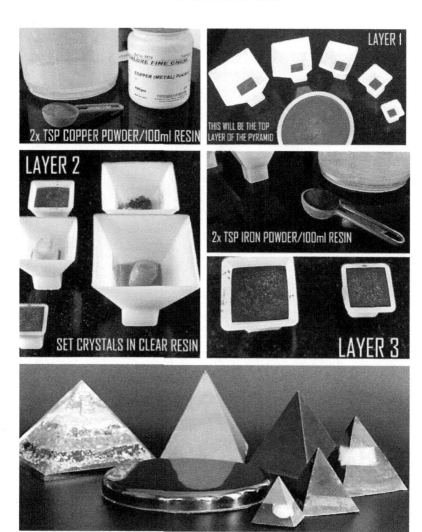

2x TSP COPPER POWDER/100ml RESIN

LAYER 1

THIS WILL BE THE TOP LAYER OF THE PYRAMID

LAYER 2

2x TSP IRON POWDER/100ml RESIN

SET CRYSTALS IN CLEAR RESIN

LAYER 3

Materials Lists

Material	Properties
Organic Insulators	
Epoxy Resin	Durable compound, sets firm, doesn't degrade over time
Paraffin Wax	Pliable, less noxious than resin, allows for moldable forms *not heat-resistant
Beeswax	Pliable, chemical-free, moldable compound *not heat resistant
Latex Paint	Liquid, can be used to coat any surface

Inorganic Metals	
Aluminum	Reflection and protection. Planet: *Mercury*, Element: *Air*
Iron	Deflects negativity, iron strength, grounding. Planet: *Mars*, Element: *Fire*
Bismuth	Transformation, visualization. Planet: *Uranus*, Element: *Air*
Copper	Conducts spiritual energy. Planet: *Venus*, Element: *Earth &Water*

Silver	Physical healing, yin energy, intuition &psychic power, divine feminine. Planet: *Moon*, Element: *Water*
Gold	Health, wealth, growth, vitality, prosperity, yang, divine masculine. Planet: *Sun*, Element: *Fire*
Titanium	Strength, stability, imperviousness. Planet: *Saturn*, Element: *Ether*

Secondary Ingredients	
Agate	Inner stability
Amazonite	Truth and courage
Amber	Protection, preservation of youth
Amethyst	Inner peace and creativity
Aquamarine	Soothing, go-with-the-flow
Azurite	Mental and emotional clarity
Bloodstone	Courage, strength and endurance
Carnelian	Fertility, creativity, taking action
Celestite	Divine power, higher consciousness
Citrine	Willpower, prosperity
Dolomite	Centering, grounding

Fluorite	Mental clarity and focus
Garnet	Spiritual protection
Jade	Longevity and wisdom
Jasper	Wholeness and healing
Kyanite	Reflect negative energy
Labradorite	Lucid dreaming
Malachite	Natural strength and protection
Moonstone	Healing, balance, intuition
Muscovite	Problem solving, connection to subconscious
Nephrite	Increase energy
Obsidian	Shadow self, self - reflection
Onyx	Facing fear, embracing personal power
Opal	Overall healing and wellbeing
Pearl	Wisdom and wealth
Pyrite	Shielding and blocking
Quartz	Purification, transformation
Sunstone	Light, warmth, love
Shungite	Environmental protection
Tanzanite	Divine healing, spiritual strength
Turquoise	Comfort, health protection
Topaz	Love, higher purpose, good fortune

Tertiary elements	
Tensor Ring	Stabilizes the bio-electric field, generates infinite subtle energy
Mobius Coil	Chaotic energy generation (must be stabilized with a crystal)
Copper Spirals	Elemental energy channeling
See the chapter on resonant frequency for charging secondary and tertiary elements.	

Chembuster

To make a Chembuster, you will need a lot more materials, including a bucket, metal pipes and at least 6 double-terminated crystals. Croft also suggests using a Cubit coil or similar in the base.

- 2 gallon bucket
- 6 x 12" pipe lengths (1" diameter)
- 6 x end caps
- 6 x couplers
- 6 x 5' pipe lengths
- 3 x plywood spacers

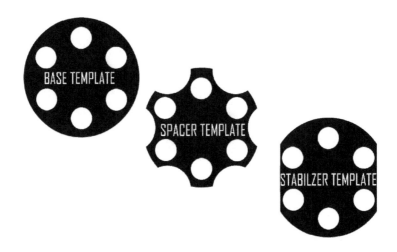

Instructions

- Before you begin construction, prepare your 3 spacing templates to fit your pipes and bucket.
- Pour the first layer of orgone-matrix material about 1.5" deep, adding a cubit coil or tensor ring and 4 crystals oriented to match the 4 compass points. This will be the base of the Chembuster. Leave to cure.
- Place the 12" sections of pipe in the first spacer.
- After placing 1 crystal in each pipe, fix the end caps to the pipes and seal with tape.
- Set the pipes and spacer into the bucket
- Pour the second layer of orgone-matrix material, adding in extra elements as required
- Slide the temporary spacer over the top of the pipes to keep them aligned while the resin cures

- Once the resin is cured, remove the temporary spacer, add the pipe connectors and join the 5' pipe lengths
- Fit the final spacer over the top end of the pipes to maintain the upward alignment.

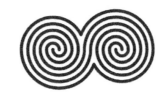

CHAPTER SIX

EXPERIMENTS FROM THE ORGONE MATRIX

Reich measured the charge of Orgone by recording the discharge time of an electroscope under specific conditions. The quantitative measure is defined as 1 org relative to the time period of the discharge. However, this method of measurement is complex and unreliable because of the prerequisite conditions. Orgone can be considered a proto-physical energy therefore it is believed that its effects can be observed in a more practical manner by its interactions with living matter. Energy-sensitive people are able to feel the effects of a good piece of orgonite the moment they come into its range. For the less sensitive among us, there are some simple tests you can do to see how effective your orgonite is. These experiments don't need any special measuring equipment, it is a simple matter of patience and observation. A quick search online will lead to videos of similar experiments, as well as some slightly more advanced tests that measure the ionisation potential of orgonite or how it affects the charge in a body or an object.

There are electronic instruments for sale online which purport to measure the life energy of any living thing and thus enable you to measure the effectiveness of your Orgone devices. These experimental life-energy meters are based on the modified instruments that Wilhelm Reich had used in his experiments to measure the presence of Orgone in live beings and various types of matter by using electrode plates, but thanks to advances in technology they are much smaller than the high-voltage induction coils used in the original machines. These are different to regular EMF meters as they respond only to "living" energy and not electromagnetic or static electric charges. Other popular methods of testing include psychic observation and dowsing, as well as the following outcomes-based experiments.

Below are the tests that you will be able to do immediately once you have your orgonite:

- **Ice Experiment**
- **Garden Experiment**
- **Entropy Experiment**

What is amazing about these tests is that they relate to the primary functions of Orgone. You will see in the ice experiment how Orgone creates a more geometric structure in materials around it, in the garden experiment how it promotes healthy growth in living things and the entropy experiment shows how a strong flow of Orgone slows down the process of decay. The best test to see the atmospheric impact of orgone-matrix materials is done with a Chembuster, which has a more powerful and pointed effect.

Ice Experiment

For this you will need two identical containers filed with the same amount of water from the same source and one piece of orgonite. The orgonite does not need to be of a specific size or shape, however a flat disk such as a charging plate or Towerbuster will be the easiest to use. Clear out enough space in the freezer so the two water containers can sit at the same level with space around them. Place the orgonite directly beneath one of the containers and simply observe what happens once the water has frozen. Most people report that the Orgone-charged water forms a vortex-like pattern once frozen. In some cases, the upward spiral of Orgone energy is so strong that the ice forms a projection out of the container.

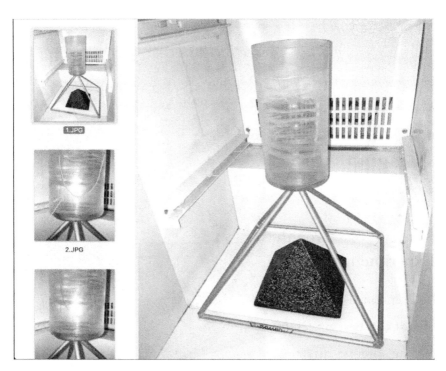

Pyramid Experiment by akaidatv

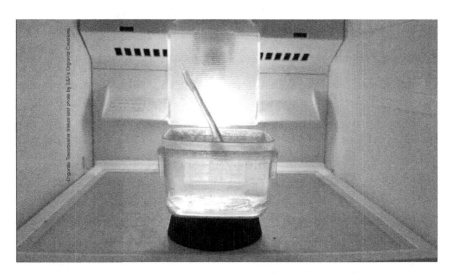

Ice pillar forming in an experiment by S&A's Orgone Creations

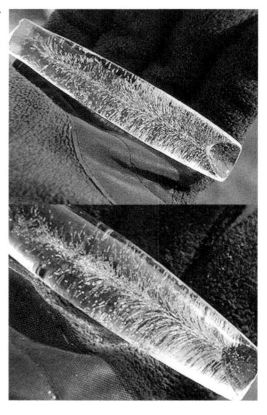

This image shows the pattern of ice formed inside a Chembuster pipe. The indentation at the lower end is from the crystals protruding from the orgone matrix base.

Garden Growth Experiment

As mentioned previously, one of the best places to put an orgone-attracting device is somewhere with a lot of sunlight and fresh air, so a garden is perfect. Some people simply scatter the orgonite pieces around among the plants, others bury them in the earth near the roots. Gardeners that grow fruit and vegetables report fantastic results in the size and taste of their produce grown with orgonite compared to those without, but its effects are also obvious with flowers and ornamental houseplants.

To test your orgonite outdoors, make sure you have a section that can be divided into two equal beds with the same quality of soil and same amount of sun exposure, so that one section can be used as your control. Plant the same plants in each bed, simply adding one or more pieces of orgonite to the part you have chosen for your experiment. For the best results, give both sections the same amount of water each day and use a measuring stick to track your plants' growth on a weekly basis. This test can also be done if you have two similar houseplants to work with.

An indoor test can also be done by sprouting seeds or beans. Again, it is important to set up an identical control system so you can compare your results. The quickest test you can do is to sprout a bean in a dark cupboard or box, simply wrap a bean or seed in dampened paper towel and place it in a cool, dark place, sprinkling fresh water on it daily to keep the towel moist. One should be placed on top of an orgone charging disk, or enclosed with a pyramid.

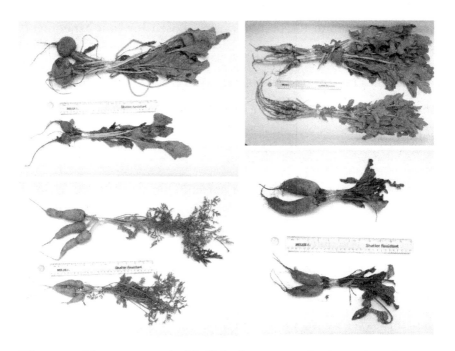

These vegetables were grown by Mr P barker as a result of an informal orgonite gardening trial organised by Mark bennett in Brighton, UK. The larger vegetables were all harvested from the orgone-enriched garden.

Entropy Experiment

Orgone energy is described as being negentropic, meaning that it counteracts decay or entropy. Be warned that this experiment does require letting some organic matter start to go rotten, so make sure you have an appropriate place to try it out and don't end up creating a health hazard. Citrus fruits are ideal for this experiment, as they naturally contain pretty good preservatives and tend to dry out rather than decompose. For this you need a flattened disk or charging plate, so you can place one piece of fruit on top for the duration of the experiment, while the other is left on a regular plate or coaster. After the first week you will be able to feel the difference in moisture content (Orgone slows the rate of water evaporation) and after a month you will see a visible difference in the rind of the two fruits. If you're curious, you can then cut the fruits in half to see how they have each decomposed. Please note that neither of them are good to eat at this point, it is simply to create a clearer picture of the effects of Orgone energy and why some people choose to keep orgonite in the fridge.

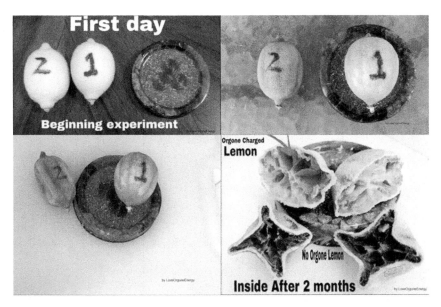

Image via Love Orgone Energy YouTube Channel

Atmospheric Experiment

The Chembuster is notorious for the "blue hole effect" that occurs in clouds, which seem to form spiral patterns and disintegrate in direct correspondence with the direction and position of the device. As you can see in the image below, the effect also occurs with vapor trails, geoengineered or otherwise. Interestingly, in Reich's descriptions of an Orgone-positive atmosphere he notes that condensation from airplanes lingers for much longer in the presence of POR than DOR. It is through the later interpretations of cosmic Orgone hypotheses that the idea of modifying a Cloudbuster to dissolve Chemtrails transpired.

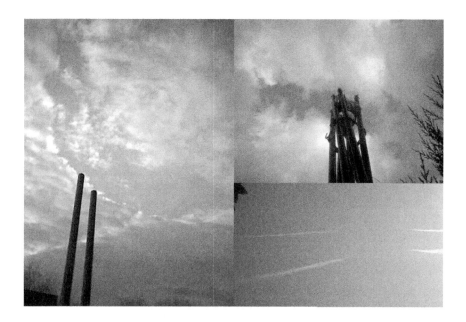

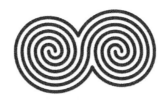

CHAPTER SEVEN

RADIATION: DOES ORGONITE REALLY PROTECT YOU?

One of the most popular ways that orgonite, Orgonium and similar products are marketed online is as radiation blocking devices. Unfortunately, it has not been proven to be any more effective at blocking EMF emissions from Wi-Fi routers than any other solid lump of matter. To help you assess the possibilities of working with orgone matrix materials, this chapter and the following section will provide explanations for some of the ambiguous scientific claims that are made about them. First, we'll be taking a look at what constitutes radiation, why some radiation is considered harmful, and Reich's ideas about its interaction with Orgone energy.

Right now, you are sloshing around in electron soup. You are electron soup. Sometimes those electrons get wildly excited because they are being irradiated, which simply means the sun is sending out abundant little packets of energy in the form of light, or photons, and you and your electrons are in the way, so you absorb them. If the weather is appropriate, take a moment to go outside, or sit next to a window and feel the warm glow of sunlight on your skin. That feeling is radiation and you are exposed to it all the time. Luckily, we have evolved under the sun so we can handle quite a lot of exposure to its radiation. In fact, if we don't expose ourselves to it often enough, we get very miserable and even physically ill. Thankfully, our atmosphere is astonishingly good at making sure none of the really deadly stuff gets through, which leaves us free to wander around outside with little to worry about other than a sunburn.

There are many different ways that radiation and matter can interact, some of them extremely harmful and others rather beneficial. For the most part, scientists think they have figured out what levels of radiation the organic beings that inhabit this planet can tolerate and so we find ourselves no longer subject only to the elemental energy of our environment, but a multitude of man-made emissions as well. Like quantized light, these come in a variety of particles and waves. The most obvious form of environmental pollution is the smog and smoke that lingers in the wake of the industrial revolution and its modern cousin — nuclear waste. The less obvious and still somewhat controversial idea is that of "clogging up the airwaves." A pollutant is described by the National Geographic society as something that damages the air, water or land.

In a Britannica article, Jerry A Nathanson expands on this by describing it as *"the addition of any substance or any form of energy to the environment at a rate faster than it can be dispersed, diluted, decomposed, recycled, or stored in some harmless form."* This includes sound and light pollution, radioactivity and heat emissions.

If one is a strict adherent of the materialistic universe theory, then one could quite easily trust that all of the technology we see popping up around us is carefully calibrated to adhere to certain safety standards. These standards are, of course, set by strict adherents of the material universe theory. Those who perceive the existence of more subtle forms of energy are not as easily convinced that radiation interacts with the causal body as predictably as it does in the physical realms. Since we are so deeply entrenched in the age of information, it would be easy enough to find a paper written by someone with the appropriate letters behind their name to confirm or deny whatever it is you wish to believe in. When it comes to electromagnetic field (EMF) exposure, there are a variety of opinions- however, the overarching one is that low-level (non-ionizing) radiation is not harmful to humans.

Because we exist under a continual source of high-level ultraviolet radiation (the sun), human skin is pretty good at blocking or absorbing radiation before it can get to our other vital organs, where it may cause undesired effects. This is part of the reason it's generally considered not to be harmful – if the skin blocks high-level radiation, low-level radiation shouldn't be a problem, right? Well, considering that even the WHO classifies certain wavelengths as "possibly carcinogenic to humans", many scientists posit articles suggesting that more studies need to be done without any conflict of interest.

The main argument against the potential damage caused by low level radiation is that the forces are not strong enough to displace electrons, which is the feature that makes high level radiation/ photon energy so powerful. While some scientists claim that constant ELF and EMF exposure can't be bad because of the negligible thermal effects, plenty of other scientists are calling for further study of the non-thermal effects, which could be linked to changes in the immune system and circadian rhythm, as well as electrical and chemical communication in the body. A particular study by Magda Havas, B.Sc., Ph.D. highlights that "free radicals can and do cause cancer and non-ionizing radiation can and does increase free radicals."

Free radicals are molecules containing oxygen with an odd number of electrons, meaning they can react easily with other molecules and start off chain reactions of chemical processes in the body. Oxidation reactions can be both beneficial and harmful, so antioxidants that help to stabilize free radicals and lower their reactivity help to maintain balance within the body. Oxidative stress occurs when there is disharmony between the two and not enough antioxidants are present to prevent free radicals from damaging vital proteins and DNA. This can contribute to an alarming array of diseases including diabetes, Parkinson's, cardiovascular disease and other inflammatory conditions. What we do know for a fact contributes to illness and disease is stress, poor sleep, and poor diet. According to a study done in Norway, workers in any job that work the night shift were more likely to develop cancer than those with prolonged exposure to low-level radiation, but what does that mean for a society that stays up all night, glued to their electronic devices?

In the year 2000, when mobile phones were becoming prevalent among the general population, a study highlighted that children are more conductive than adults (due to higher moisture and ionic content) and the effects of RF could affect their nervous system development more significantly, but studies are not done on children so the true effects of exposing their developing brains and bodies to radiation can be discussed only anecdotally, which of course holds very little standing in the scientific community where empirical evidence is king. Many people feel that the rise in behavioral disorders in children is because of the constant electromagnetic disruptions.

In the spectrum of radiofrequency, ultraviolet, x-rays and y-rays are ionizing forms of radiation known as high level radiation or microwave radiation. Low-level radiation has two subcategories: ELF and EMF. ELF stands for extremely low frequency and includes wavelengths from 3 – 300Hz. The research investigating the potential damage that can be caused by ELF radiation is described as "controversial," which basically means that even the WHO and OSHA in the US aren't entirely sure. However, they seem to be erring on the side of publishing studies from the early 1990s, long before 48.37% of the world's population owned smartphones and the advent of Wi-Fi.

Let's take a look at the radiation spectrum:

NON-IONIZING:

•ELF

•Radio Frequency

•Microwaves

•Visible light

Includes power lines, Bluetooth, MRI, mobile phones, microwaves, computers, etc.

IONIZING:

•UV

•X-RAY

•GAMMA

Includes sunlight, x-ray machines, radioactive waste.

In general, you'd be hard-pressed to find a report from any health organization that doesn't come with heavy disclaimers stating that much more research is needed. For example, here is a statement from the United States' Occupational Safety and Health Administration:

"The issue of extremely low frequency (ELF) biological effects is very controversial. Research has focused on possible carcinogenic, reproductive, and neurological effects. Other suggested health effects include cardiovascular, brain and behavior, hormonal and immune system changes."

In light of this, it's easy to assume that if some (however minor or seemingly unrelated effects) are manifesting in the physical body, that some potential harm is taking place in the energetic body. But since the concept of energy and life force is considered "bunk" by "serious" scientists, it is nearly impossible to investigate whether or not the primordial energy is affected by man-made frequencies. According to the one man who tried to quantify biophysical energy, the negative effects of continual exposure have been measured and declared dangerous. That man was Wilhelm Reich.

In his research from the 1950s, he describes a phenomenon known as DOR-sickness, which occurs when there has been a disruption to the natural flow of energy (via nuclear or other forms of radiation). The symptoms of DOR-sickness bear a lot of similarities to the effects recorded by those who claim to be hypersensitive to electromagnetic radiation - they include:

- General fatigue
- Emotional distress
- Random outbursts of hate/aggression
- Persisting nausea, diarrhea

- Pressure in the head, chest and arms
- Difficulty breathing, feeling that there is not enough oxygen
- Unhealthy pallor, dull and glazed eyes -
- Extreme thirst
- Tachycardia, heart problems

A lot of these symptoms are also reported by those who work in offices, which are more often than not crammed full of fluorescent lighting, high-powered computers and bright monitors, wireless Internet, mobile phones and an authoritarian hierarchy that discourages personal expression and innovation. In many such buildings, windows are not designed to be opened and no fresh air is available to circulate. In the northern hemisphere it is common for people to go days without seeing natural light during the winter months. This is what Reich meant when he said that the human sickness is inherited from society. There is no single element that can be blamed, so studies based on a single element will rarely reveal the truth. Perhaps on its own, continual exposure to EMF is not so bad, but the circumstances under which it happens and the increasing inability to escape from these environments is proving to be detrimental.

Programming Frequencies

"Each celestial body, in fact each and every atom, produces a particular sound on account of its movement, its rhythm or vibration. All these sounds and vibrations form a universal harmony in which each element, while having it's own function and character, contributes to the whole." - Pythagoras

The idea of the electric universe opens up a myriad of new ways to perceive and interact with reality based on resonance and frequency. Most people have heard of the Schumann resonances, which refer to a range of extremely low frequency (ELF) global electromagnetic resonances that occur as a result of the planet's ionic or electrical activity, which might sound complex but really just means lightning charges affecting the atmospheric conditions. These frequencies have been used to monitor Earth's climate conditions and could potentially teach us how to predict natural events such as earthquakes, or even to learn about the ionospheres of other planets which could reveal more about extraterrestrial phenomena.

7.83 Hz is considered to be the fundamental frequency of Earth. The range of resonance fluctuates all the time, but they generally fall within the same range of frequencies that can be measured in humans, which suggest a harmony between our vibration and the planet's. Many people are interested in how this background resonance affect the human body and consciousness, particularly because of its correlation with the frequencies of brainwaves during different states of consciousness.

In physics there is a concept called *entrainment*, which means that two oscillating bodies of different frequencies will eventually match themselves to vibrate in harmony. This is where the idea of being "in sync" comes from and it happens on a macro scale (humans synchronized to planet - biochronology, circadian rhythms etc.) and also on a micro scale (brainwave synchronization).

The neural activity and frequencies that are present in different states of consciousness are classified into five groups: Delta, Theta, Alpha, Beta and Gamma. Through entrainment, the brain can become engaged with altered states of consciousness at will.

The lowest frequency (0-4Hz) are Delta waves, which occur in deep, dreamless sleep or unconscious states. Theta Waves (4-8Hz) occur at the first phase of sleep or in deep meditation, the gap between waking and dreaming where vivid mental imagery can appear. Alpha waves (8-12Hz) comprise the "default" waking mode of consciousness, passive and relaxed awareness and coordination. Beta waves (12-30Hz) reflect a highly active brain state linked with information processing, focused mental activity and even heightened states like anxiety or the fight or flight response. Gamma waves (30-100Hz) are associated with bilateral information processing, integrating both hemispheres of the brain simultaneously. This is often linked to the idea of "higher consciousness" because it changes the scope of perception and awareness.

Since these waves and frequencies are simply electromagnetic vibrations, it is easy enough to replicate them at will. The most popular way to access these frequencies is through music and frequency generators, which are the core component of Radionics-type devices (as produced by Raymond Rife and Karl Welz.) The idea of using sound vibrations for healing is found in many ancient cultures that used chanting and music, either in ritual or medicine and was first documented in a way that is familiar to modern science by Pythagoras.

Here are some commonly referenced frequencies for healing, meditation and heightened states of awareness:

- ≈ 0.30 - 0.15 Hz: Mood elevator, against depressive states of mind
- ≈ 0.9 Hz: Feeling of euphoria
- ≈ 1 Hz: Pituitary stimulation, general harmony and balance
- ≈ 3 Hz: Increased reaction time
- ≈ 3.4 Hz: Sound sleep
- ≈ 3.5 Hz: Feeling of Oneness with everything, language learning improved enhancement of receptivity
- ≈ 4 Hz: Extrasensory perception, remote viewing, strengthens memory, physical stimulation, faster recovery after physical training
- ≈ 4.5 Hz: Dream states, shamanic consciousness, vivid imagery
- ≈ 4.6 Hz: Emotional impulsivity
- ≈ 4.9 Hz: Introspection, relaxation, meditation, deep sleep
- ≈ 5 Hz: Learning, unusual problem solving enhanced
- ≈ 5.8 Hz: Diminishes fear, works against being scattered
- ≈ 6.0 Hz: Long term memory stimulation
- ≈ 6.5 Hz: Accelerated learning
- ≈ 6.88 Hz: Inner balance and calmness
- ≈ 7.0 Hz: Mental and astral projection, telekinesis, mind projection
- ≈ 7.5 Hz: Creativity, inward focus, discovery of "purpose" in life, creative thought facilitates contact with spirit guides; facilitates

entry into meditation, lucid dreaming.

≈ 7.83 Hz: Earth Resonance, grounding, "Schumann Resonance," counteracts mind control, accelerated learning, more tolerance of stressful situations

≈ 8.0 Hz: Past life regression, hypnotic states, reduces stress, diminishes states of anxiety, strong relaxation, connection with past lives enhanced

≈ 8.3 Hz: Mental imagery, clairvoyance, ESP

≈ 10 Hz: Seratonin release

≈ 10.5 Hz: Heart chakra

≈ 12 Hz: Throat chakra

≈ 12.3 Hz: Powers of visualization

≈ 13 Hz: Ajna Chakra, powers of visualization and conceptualization

≈ 15.4 Hz: Cortex, intelligence

≈ 16.4 Hz: Crown Chakra, Transcendence

≈ 20 Hz: Overcoming fatigue, energizing

≈ 22.0 Hz: Astral traveling

≈ 25 Hz: Self-confidence, confidence of victory in sports

≈ 33 Hz: Christ consciousness, hypersensitivity, Pyramid frequency

≈ 35 Hz: Awakening, balance of chakras

≈ 38 Hz: Endorphin release

≈ 40 Hz: Evolution when problem solving in fearful situations, leadership especially where fast action is required

≈ 55 Hz: Tantra, kundalini

≈ 62 Hz: Feeling of physical vigor

≈ 70 Hz: Mental and astral projection

≈ 80 Hz: Awareness and control of right direction

≈ 98 Hz: Dan Tien

≈ 108 Hz: Total knowing

≈ 111 Hz: Beta endorphins and cell regeneration

≈ 126.2 Hz: Sun

≈ 136.1 Hz: Sun: light, warmth, joy 140.2 Hz: Pluto: power, crisis & changes

≈ 141.2 Hz: Mercury: intellectuality, mobility

≈ 144.7 Hz: Mars: activity, energy, freedom, humor

≈ 147.8 Hz: Saturn: separation, sorrow, death

≈ 183.5 Hz: Jupiter: growth, success, justice, spirituality

≈ 194.7 Hz: Earth: stability, grounding

≈ 207.3 Hz: Uranus: spontaneity, independence, originality

≈ 211.4 Hz: Neptune: unconscious, secrets, imagination, spiritual love

≈ 221.2 Hz: Venus: beauty, love, sexuality, sensuality, harmony

≈ 247 Hz: Feeling of peacefulness

≈ 250 Hz: Elevate and revitalize

≈ 384 Hz: *Gurdjieff vibration associated with root chakra.

≈ 396 Hz: *Solfeggio - Liberating guilt and fear

≈ 417 Hz: *Solfeggio - Undoing Situations/Facilitating Change

≈ 420.8 Hz: Moon: love, sensitivity, creativity, femininity

≈ 432 Hz: Cosmic frequency, structure of the universe

≈ 494 Hz: Spiritual awakening

≈ 528 Hz: DNA healing / *Solfeggio - Transformation and Miracles

≈ 639 Hz: *Solfeggio - Connecting/Relationships

≈ 741 Hz: *Solfeggio - Expression/Solutions

≈ 794 Hz: Strong willpower

≈ 852 Hz: *Solfeggio - Returning to spiritual order

PART - III

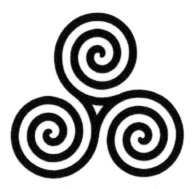

The Science of Orgonite

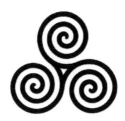

CHAPTER EIGHT

THE PHYSICS

T he two main effects that are cited as facilitating the interaction between orgonite and the Orgone field are the Casimir effect and the Piezoelectric effect. While these forces are easily observable in the traditional models of physics, it is impossible to observe in the subtle energy field because it is believed that the effects are taking place on an atomic level, changing the geometric structure of the energy itself.

Let's take a look at the Casimir effect first, as this is what is at work in orgonite, even where no quartz has been integrated. The Casimir effect is a force that emerges when two metal plates are brought into close proximity to each other. From the quantum model of the universe, we understand that particles are constantly popping in and out of existence in the "empty" spaces all around us. When the two metal plates are close enough together, there is a limit to the number and size of particles that may spontaneously appear between them. There is no such limit on the space around the plates. This imbalance results in a force that is generated between the plates, becoming so strong that it causes the plates to clamp together at which point the effect collapses and can no longer be observed.

It has been recorded that the smaller the plates get, the stronger the power of the Casimir effect. Inside the orgone matrix material are thousands of tiny metal filings acting in much the same way as the plates from the Casimir experiment, generating a force from nothing more than existing in the right arrangement within their environment. It is generally believed that this effect, when combined with the piezoelectric effect of crystals like quartz, produces a much more profound phenomenon.

Piezoelectric materials are unique in that they have the power to transform a mechanical force into an electrical charge and vice versa. The most popular application of this is in quartz watches and it works because of the geometrical atomic structure of the quartz crystal. For the effect to work, the quartz has to be cut at a certain angle that will allow compression of the octahedral grid formed by the silicon and oxygen molecules that quartz consists of. This compression creates a charge, or when the crystal receives a charge, the inverse happens and the crystalline grid compresses, causing a resultant force.

In an orgone matrix, the quartz powder is said to be able to produce a tiny charge under the constant pressure of the micro-contraction index, which is a combined result of the pressure of resin shrinking as it sets and the Casimir effect taking place between the metallic particles. Normally a sustained pressure would be ineffective, but some experts suggest that the coherent crystalline structure of the crystal polyester resin allows these forces to be maintained within the matrix material. The impulses generated by the pressurized quartz particles "polarize" DOR that is accumulated or retained in the metal-resin matrix by reforming its corrupted structure. Depending on the shape of the orgonite, the Orgone which allegedly seeks to ascend vertically, will form an upward vortex of restructured energy. In this way, orgonite acts like a transformer, or a purifier of Orgone energy, rather than just an accumulator which will amplify even the damaged or damaging forms of Orgone.

Unfortunately, material scientists disagree. In regard to the Piezoelectric effect that is said to occur when the shrinking resin compresses the quartz, scientists insist that this force would be insufficient to initiate the effect. It is even less likely that it would have a sustained effect over a prolonged period of time. Polymerization is not enough of a stress to create a distortion in the crystal that generates an electric charge, and even if it were it would require an oscillating mechanical stress, meaning a repetitive application of force. It is most likely that the amount of stress necessary to generate the effect would fracture the resin matrix and break the piece. These scientists also refer to the law of conservation of energy- that is, that energy can only be transferred from one form to another, not created or generated, so if an orgonite piece (what they would call a "static system") is said to be producing energy, according to classical science it must have come from somewhere. This is why Karl Welz's Orgone Generators need to be connected to an external current to effectively create an orgone charge.

Another false claim that seems to haunt the world of orgonite is that the resin-metal compound is capable of producing negative ions which is simply wrong, to be quite blunt. Like the other effects listed, the production of negative ions is subject to the presence of mechanical force, electrical action or radioactive decay. A quick reading of some orgone blogs will reveal plenty of information about the very real and proven benefits of negative ions, which is then spuriously linked to orgonite with no mention of how the effect is produced.

The ion charge of metals is positive, whereas the organic material is more likely to have negatively charged ions. No chemical reaction takes place between the matrix elements that are bound in close proximity to each other, but the polar ionic excitation is said to be responsible for the attraction of subtle energy. The addition of crystals is supposed to be the element that elevates the energy-attracting compound to one that is capable of quantum transmutation, using the intrinsic crystalline signature to form more coherent, higher frequency energy from corrupted or incoherent energy structures.

A lot of these egregious claims are generated from misunderstanding rather than malice and it would appear that references to principles from physics are not intended to mislead so much as create a scope of understanding about what is known about the way energy works. It is generally believed that Orgone physics takes place in higher dimensions than what we can call the 3-D physics of the material universe, so in a system that rejects the notion of etheric energy, or Orgone, it would definitely seem as though there is no "input" energy for the device to transform. However, if one shifts to Reich's model of omnipresent, permeating energy, then it leaves room for a more optimistic interpretation of the claims made about the orgone matrix.

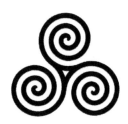

CHAPTER NINE

AN ORGONOMIC THEORY OF EVERYTHING

It has long since been determined that we live in a chaotic world, right down to the fundamental forces that shape our material environment and the interaction we have with it. The mathematical functions that describe our universe are full of paradoxes and probabilities. Beyond a certain point, scientists' attempts to create order break down, requiring an entirely new model as a frame of reference. The point at which our knowledge currently breaks down is the subatomic level. Entirely new models of thought and mathematics have been developed to quantify the effects of interactions at this level:

Quantum mechanics.

Many scientists and philosophers throughout history have held on to the notion that all interactions are taking place within a field of some description. The exact description of that field has evaded them for the better part of recorded human history. In fact, most cultures simply called it God and let the priests and sages take it from there. It exists in the ancient Asiatic traditions by the names of prana and chi. In Europe it was called aether, elan vital, even Odylic force which invokes the name of Odin in its etymology. What is common among all theories is that this living force moves within us and can be controlled by us to better support human existence.

Thanks to the advances of science and technology, today we can observe those patterns that proliferate throughout the universe on microcosmic and macro-cosmic scales. What remains implicit in these observations, is that all of these repeating patterns that obey mathematical laws are all taking place within an energy-based system, which scientists have made great efforts to quantize. This is where we get the concept of zero-point energy from, the lowest measurable amount of energy that matter can possess in a vacuum, a vibration that characterizes the nature of every element and particle. The zero-point field is a mirror of Reich's primordial, protophysical Orgone, the point at which nothing becomes something. In the same way that quantum scientists diverged from the path of classical physics, Reich was simply creating a new model to describe the phenomena that he had observed, in spite of its failure to be taken seriously among the mainstream community of scientists active at the time.

Whether or not similarities can be drawn between them, it is not necessary to describe the effects of the Orgone matrix according to classical or even quantum mechanical models, because the energy itself does not seem to be confined by such a set of parameters. The fundamental interaction taking place is the same that has been spoken of since the dawn of time - it is the yin and yang, the shiva and the shakti. In Reich's own words:

"…we were dealing with a functional process which somehow converted cosmic energy directly into a matter-like substance (E → M) and also the opposite way (M→ E). These functions were assumed to be operating below the realm of mechanical, electrical, and chemical functions as pre-atomic, sub-chemical, primordial functions of the Universe."

This means that the process taking place inside the orgone matrix is a re-polarization of fundamental energy. If you imagine the organic materials as a "pulling" force and the inorganic materials as a "pushing" force, when orgone passes through the matrix it goes through a process of chaotic deconstruction that allows it to return to its default state, much like honey resuming the shape of the honeycomb after being swirled in water. Any corruption or damage to the innate structure of Orgone can be undone by this process of attracting and repelling, using the knowledge that Reich left behind about the way different types of materials interact with Orgone.

With this understanding, the difference between Orgone Accumulators, Orgone Generators and Orgone Matrices becomes clear. The Accumulator with its limited layered structure can only condense Orgone in whatever form is currently in the atmosphere and contain it within the structure of the accumulator. The Generator requires an external power source and is supposed to be capable of both generating and restructuring Orgone. The matrix material, or orgonite, depending on whose rationale you follow, is capable of restructuring negative energy and/or attracting Orgone to an environment and projecting it outward, as opposed to the finite containment of the ORAC.

"The concepts of Orgone Accumulator and Orgone energy are considered pseudoscience according to modern science. Theoretically it is consistent in itself but inconsistent with other basic disciplines."

This quote comes from a study done by Serdar Yukseland Özgür Eroglu, in which they observed that plants in an Orgone Accumulator grew 30% longer than the plants in the control environment. In the results of the study, they are forced to acknowledge that the "pseudoscientific" subject is worthy of further investigation due to the affirmative outcomes of their experiments. This kind of genuine and objective replication of his experiments and investigation of his theories is not a privilege that Reich was afforded in his lifetime; he was perpetually frustrated by those that would denounce him without even making an attempt at disproving his work.

There is no single body or organization that can speak on behalf of science. Science is a process, not an establishment, although there are many who would have you believe otherwise. In fact, it is only the establishment that purports to present a unified voice among scientists, where in reality, science is practiced by people, who all come with their own diversity of opinions, agendas and axes to grind. Reich was neither the first nor the last to come up with a model that wasn't entirely compatible with the mainstream view, but he used the process of science to describe what he had observed.

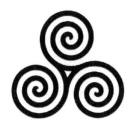

CHAPTER TEN

THE IMPORTANCE OF STRUCTURE

"If there is a God, he's a great mathematician." - PAUL DIRAC

A tomic Geometry a new theory that transcends the incoherence between quantum physics and relativity, brought about by. This is a theory that allows both concepts to be accurate, and there's room for the aetheric energy too. Imagine a combined model of particle physics and sacred geometry; this is essentially the foundation of the theory. For the concept of aether as a medium in which electromagnetic waves travel through a vacuum to be viable, it needs to fulfill a particular criterion: it must express the nature of an incompressible fluid, meaning it has a constant density throughout. This is a concept borrowed from a complex field of theoretical study known as continuum mechanics, which models the physical phenomena of matter under the assumption that it is continuously distributed and fills the entire region of space it occupies. 4D Aether theory is an adaptation of classical Ether Theory that suggests hypercubic space as the 4-D substance needed to substantiate the idea of a medium that transmits the electromagnetic waves that our reality consists of, as a cube is a Platonic solid that is capable of uniformly filling space.

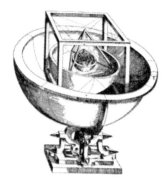

Kepler's Mysterium Cosmographicum

Using 4-D thinking to get acquainted with the concept of atomic geometry is the first step in understanding the interactions between orgone (aether) and matter, which will provide a unique framework for explaining what takes place inside the orgone-matrix. The correlation of space and time is often considered as the fourth dimension of the reality that we perceive; however, this new interpretation assigns that dimension with its own spatial characteristic, or shape. This shape has a geometry which is based on the structure of the atom itself.

The shape of time can be expressed as a Toroidal field, a point, which transforms into a circle, then collapses back into its original point, like the visualization of the field generated between the poles of a magnet. This is time, which is simply the way we measure reality changing from one moment to the next, with each new moment expressed as a point that contains within it the memories, movement and direction of the moment before.

This constant transformation and morphing of space is an enactment of the qualities of the 4th dimension: a shape that is continuously switching between two states. The Torus field is a fundamental component of understanding gravity and electromagnetism. The poles of the earth generate a Torus field that certain animal can interact with innately and humans have learned how to exploit artificially for communication, even the human aura is said to take the shape of the Torus field.

The Torus field can be seen as the energy field which essentially powers the 3-D reality which is represented in the 4th dimension as a matrix of hypercubic space, each tesseract continually changing phase to "update" reality as perceived from within the 3-D matrix. The "inner" cube represents the tangible reality that we interact with using our senses and the "outer" cube represents the unmanifest energy of matter.

Of course, we can only experience one of these endlessly switching cubes at a time and using the Planck scale, we can quantize moments of time at an atomic level within the cubic space that we inhabit. These ideas coalesce to support the idea of a quantized fractal reality.

The key to the fourth dimension is transformation and it is not only the Torus and hypercube that explain how multidimensional realities can be connected through the morphing of form, there are other shapes, for example the cross which becomes a square at a 45-degree angle, which represent the concept of inverse geometry. This is an important mechanism to describe what is happening in reality from the lowest level and predicts causality at higher levels. Geometry in this way describes reality according to two fundamental forces of the universe: expansion and contraction. If that sounds familiar, it's because this model uncovers the same premise that Wilhelm Reich observed while explaining the nature of Orgone.

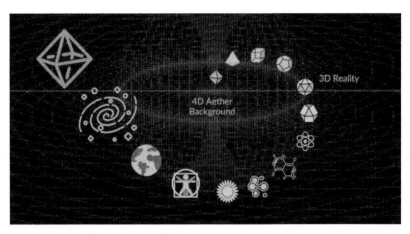

Graphic from Atomic Geometry module at in2infinity.com

The physical forms that we experience in everyday life are made up of atoms and molecules that are organized in a specific fashion and each atom can be mapped through various geometric forms that represent the manifestation of matter from an infinite fourth-dimensional background energy. Using Geo-quantum mechanics, Colin can explain the atomic blueprint formed by the configuration of electrons within a cube of empty space, which predicts with a new accuracy the atomic radius of stable elements. Electrons are often vaguely depicted as buzzing around atoms, but they actually appear in structures that are like a matrix. Each pattern can be ascribed a geometric shape and the forms of different elements maintain a logical ratio according to their periodic sequence.

Everything that you're experiencing in reality is either electric or magnetic energy. Electromagnetism makes up light waves and light waves make up a large part of the thing we're experiencing as the energy that flows through the universe. These two energies, electricity and magnetism, are the same phenomena but observed from different perspectives. Relativity encompasses the idea that energy and mass are equivalent and transmutable, as depicted in Einstein's famous equation, $E=mc^2$.

Matter is defined as that which occupies space and has mass, so this theory posits an equivalence of energy and matter, at least mathematically. This means that you can choose to view phenomena in different ways, imagining, for example, that a light wave is still, while the electron moves through it, or conversely that the electron is static and it is the light wave that is in motion. This particular example is nearly always viewed from the perspective where the light wave is in motion, but Colin Power suggests that the key to understanding Orgone energy is to observe the electromagnetic system from the perspective of the slower moving energy, the electron. Orgone energy is a slow-moving energy, so it bears more similarity to the qualities of electrons, which are present in all of matter. For that reason, Orgone is considered to be an energy of matter.

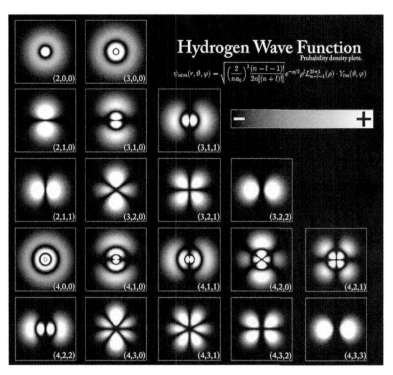

Wavefunctions of the hydrogen atom predicted by Schrödinger's equation

The De Broglie wavelength of electrons describes the wave properties of matter and Schrodinger's wave equations predict the behavior of charged atoms. This was revealed in an experiment in which a hydrogen atom was charged up with energy, which formed various wave patterns around the atom depending on the amount of energy applied. What this shows you is that the space of probability around the hydrogen atom is geometric and being constantly filled with energy which creates a quantized effect. Thus, Colin has deduced that Orgone energy is not a quantized phenomenon but a resonance, which only comes into effect when it's filling space, which has a geometry. Reality can only be quantized in such a way when the energy that powers it is filling material space.

There's a lot more to this theory, but it supports the idea of Orgone as an etheric resonance. Orgonite is designed to exploit the interaction of resonance and matter to amplify the amount of energy that becomes available. When you examine the atomic structure of the organic-inorganic combination of elements inside an orgone matrix, it is revealed that they possess a coherent geometry which affects the dimensional space available to be filled by the resonant energy. Electrons in metallic elements are found at higher density, which means more energy is absorbed in electron-electron collisions. In an insulator, like carbon-based compounds or quartz, the electrons regain nearly all of their energy because they are colliding with ions instead.

When embedded in a crystalline solid, an atom experiences multiple axes and no set direction. This means that in a complex matrix structure, entirely different quantum geometries are forming based on the interaction of the separate materials. Although this theory is still in its speculative stages, it would suggest that the geometry formed by the quantum interactions of orgone-matrix materials with resonant energy allows for a more complete saturation of space with energy.

Shape and form take on paramount importance when you realize that Orgone is the charging of the geometric spaces within a substance. Science has focused all of its attention on measuring energy, but has never taken a step back to see that energy acts within the parameters of geometry. Geometry is what defines the structure of things. Without geometry, there can be only chaos. The idea of life and consciousness is that they are that which has emerged from the chaos to create order.

PART - IV

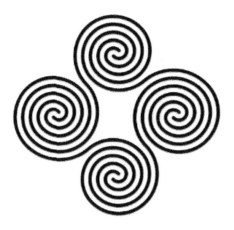

Past, Present, Future

"No President, Academy, Court of Law, Congress or Senate on this earth has the knowledge or power to decide what will be the knowledge of tomorrow."

-Wilhelm Reich [Contact with Space]

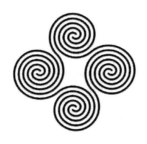

CHAPTER ELEVEN

REICH: PROFILING THE PARIAH

"I shall list my most important discoveries and views, in abbreviated form:

- *The electrical nature of sexuality*
- *The tension-charge formula*
- *Orgone radiation*
- *Bion development from cooked, prepared matter*
- **The Cancer Biopathy*
- *The self-decomposition of the human organism due to poor breathing, which serves to repress instincts*
- *The T-bacilli as a product of self-decomposition and incipient cancer biopathy*
- *The radiating SAPA bions*
- *Vegetotherapy*
- *The sociology of sex"*

-From American Odyssey, a compilation of Reich's personal notes edited by Mary Boyd-Higgins

A t a time when academics and professionals were expected to stay within the limits of their respective fields and there was little room for crossover, Wilhelm Reich was a very unique figure. He defied this construct and expanded his studies to include law, medicine, psychoanalysis, politics and philosophy, all of which contributed to the holistic model of his observations and his determination to prove, with quantifiable evidence, that a fundamental force of life energy not only exists, but could be manipulated too.

Reich was born at the very end of the 19th Century in a part of the Austro-Hungarian Empire called Galicia, an area which falls within Ukrainian borders today. His somewhat troubled childhood has been extensively recorded biographically as well as in Reich's own writings. Through some of Reich's own techniques of analysis, which bear some resemblance to today's critical and intersectional theories, many have speculated on how his early life experiences shaped the man he would become. Both of his parents had died before he reached adulthood and like many others, he was forced to endure the frontlines of the first world war. Reich wrote about the profound effects the war had on his psyche. Like many intellectuals, he was appalled by the display of man as machine, acting only in accordance with direct instruction, witnessing rank after rank of bodies purged of their humanity.

The destruction and poverty at the end of the war left him with nowhere to go but Vienna, in the hopes of finding an education and a career. It is said that he initially hoped to study Law, but instead sought to pursue a career as a physician. Freud and the Vienna Psychoanalytic Society were enjoying the peak of their academic significance in their attempts to understand Libido and neurosis, through a series of lectures in Sexology, which the student Reich was able to attend. The topic so fascinated him, that he changed his own vocational aspirations and under the mentorship of Freud himself, became one of the youngest members ever to be admitted to the association of psychoanalysts. Using his background in medicine, Reich worked hard to prove the link between physical and mental health, which were treated as entirely separate fields of study in the early 20th century. Wilhelm Reich could have been, like Freud, one of the "grandfathers" of the 21st century. There are many who do consider him to be a luminary, but unfortunately still more consider him to be a quack and a charlatan. In hindsight, using those same analytical skills that Reich himself is responsible for pioneering, is obvious when and why Reich began his descent from respectability.

In his first book, *The Function of the Orgasm*, Reich revealed his understanding that the body is energetic in its physical and non-physical functioning. The orgasm's function, per Reich, is to facilitate total relaxation and release of energy, bringing body and mind back into a state of harmonious equilibrium. In his own words:

"The elimination of the sexual stasis by the orgastic discharge of the biological excitation removes every kind of neurotic manifestation."

In a healthy organism, the orgasm is the culmination of this increased charge in a release that serves to remove built up tensions that can go on to cause physical and mental debilitations if left unchecked. Even when Freud abandoned his theory of the Libido as a measurable force, Reich understood that we live in an energetic universe, and that the primary mode of energetic expression is sexual – the force of procreation or reproduction. Reich saw this aspiration towards homeostasis as a series of energetic transactions, which he termed "Sex Economy." The idea of expansion and contraction was paramount to his understanding of the energetic economy of the body; a healthy "orgastic potency" as he called it, meant a strong charge of flowing, expansive energy in the body, symbolic of openness and fluidity. A diminished potency was synonymous with a contracted, withdrawn and tightening energy that was evident in sickly and neurotic individuals. This term would later be changed to "orgonomic potential" once the scope of Reich's study broadened to include all functions of nature.

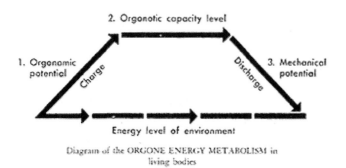

Diagram of the ORGONE ENERGY METABOLISM in living bodies

Reich went on to develop the concept of "armoring" to describe the way people try to protect themselves from stress in their environments. He observed the way people carry stiffness and tension in their bodies, "hardening" themselves as a result of psychic discomfort. In a work titled Character Analysis, he introduced the art of Vegetotherapy which was a complete departure from the norms of psychoanalytic therapy because it involved physical interaction with the patient. At the time, the vegetative nervous system was the name given to what is now referred to as the autonomic nervous system – the parts of our body that run without our conscious control – and Reich found immense value in teaching people how to interact with their bodies at this level. Inspired as he was by Freud, Reich understood the implication of repression of natural instinct and sought to relieve people of the torment caused by the repression of their sexuality, their anger, their grief, or any other emotion or issue. In his somewhat controversial therapeutic practices, he would sometimes quite literally prod and poke his clients into expressing their visceral rage and anger, allowing them an orgasmic level of release of repressed instinct or emotion.

The more time he spent with his patients and research, the more aware Reich became of the socio-political influence on the formation of our characters. At various points throughout human history, society has upheld varying standards of social conduct and interaction. In the words of his student, Charles Kelly: "Reich saw quite clearly that the sickness of man was socially or culturally transmitted." Attitudes towards sexual behavior are normally very indicative of the rules that govern a particular society and in the late 1920s and early 1930s, liberated sexual expression was considered very much an undesirable, Bohemian trait by the zealous National Socialist Party that was rising to power in Germany, where Reich carried out much of his work.

Looking at the bigger picture, Reich could see how the constructs of society affect the health of its participants, so when he published a booklet (The Mass-Psychology of Fascism) explaining as much, he suddenly found himself very much out of favor among his academic circles that had aligned themselves, presumably out of self-preservation, with the Nazis. Aside from advocating for a more liberated society, Reich already had two strikes against his name, the first simply by being born to Jewish parents, their decision to raise him without religion notwithstanding, and the second being his open membership of the Communist Party. In spite of his criticisms of the movement, Reich was ultimately a Marxist and this in combination with his avant-garde approach to therapy ended in his expulsion from the psychoanalytic society where he had once been earmarked for greatness. The Communist Party was banned the day after Hitler took power, and Reich fled to London while his "depraved" ideas burned in Berlin.

While in London, Reich was able to secure himself a working visa for Norway where he would go on to continue his research. The work he was doing at this time would change everything that he thought he knew about the universe. Due to restrictions on his visa, he was unable to practice as a psychotherapist, so Reich turned his attention to the biological experiments that would help explain some of the theories he had been using in his psychoanalytic work. In an attempt to better understand his own theory of Sex Economy, Reich wanted to quantify the energy he thought of as bio-electricity and so he used electromagnetic plates to measure the charge on the skin during states of arousal, proving that the body becomes more charged as sexual stimulation and excitement increases, whereas the charge decreases with anxiety and unpleasant emotions. He noticed that the energy he was measuring expressed itself very differently to electromagnetic energy, moving much slower with a longer wavelength and wondered if the same processes could be observed in simpler life forms.

This was when he discovered bions, which would be the precursor to all we know about Orgone energy today. Having discovered that certain chemicals cause responses in the autonomic nervous system that aligned with his theory of expansion (parasympathetic engagement) and contraction (sympathetic nervous system engagement), Reich embarked on a study of biochemistry in tandem with his theory of bioenergy. He was observing sterilized solutions of inorganic matter under a microscope, when he noticed two things he wasn't expecting: movement and light. He believed he was seeing organic life emerging from disintegrating sterile matter, which would mean that there is some vital life force at play, capable of permeating and infusing matter with its energy. He wondered if this life force was the same energy which gathers and builds in human bodies when they reach peaks of excitement and so revisited his earlier work, looking for ways to correlate the new findings. What Reich was able to conclude, was that there is a field of energy which all of life is experiencing constant interactions with. Using the same root as the word orgasm, for indeed orgasm is the beginning of life, Reich called this energy Orgone. He noted that when a cell or a body is having a healthy charge of Orgone, a radiant blue aura forms around it which is visible under sufficient magnification or contact photography.

Astonished by his discovery, Reich immediately sought validation from his peers, however he was met with a most extreme disappointment. Professor Leiv Kreyberg, declared that he had simply failed to properly sterilize his solutions or equipment and what he had witnessed in his microscope was nothing more than airborne bacteria multiplying in the solution. When asked to reproduce the experiment or suggest better control conditions, the scientist summarily dismissed Reich and his efforts. Reich was not deterred and continued to apply his new knowledge to helping people as best he could; like any conscientious man of medicine, Reich was interested in what causes cancer, so that it might be cured and prevented. Eventually, it would be this intention that landed him in jail.

Professor Kreyberg used his influence to prevent Reich from obtaining cancer samples to experiment with and together with a group of religiously and morally aligned peers, made a point of denouncing Reich's work without ever attempting to disprove it. This was of critical consequence when Reich was being considered for funding from the Rockefeller Foundation, an organization that essentially uses its immense financial power to define what is and is not valid science, even today. What followed for Reich in Oslo was a bitter campaign of defamation that was run in newspapers to color the public opinion of the "mad scientist" they were harboring. In part, he was denigrated for his lack of adherence to scientific norms, but in truth it was Reich's progressive politics and sex research that sparked moral outrage. It was eventually agreed that they would not go so far as to turn him over to the Gestapo, but he was barred from renewing his work permit and it was strongly implied that he finds another country in which to continue his efforts.

Although he had lost credibility among state-associated scientists, Reich was not without sympathy and several people saw value in his work and encouraged him to continue. There were very few options for a man in his position and so he found himself, serendipitously, on the last voyage to America before the outbreak of the second world war. In his new laboratory, a giant ranch in the state of Maine he called Orgonon, Reich continued to speculate on his earlier discoveries and advance new theories, financing his research with funds that he accrued through reestablishing his psychoanalytic practice and taking on patients.

It wasn't until 1940 that Reich invented the Orgone Accumulator and used it to help further his understanding of the properties of Orgone energy itself, as well as how it could be implemented therapeutically.

The cancer-related experiments that he had been unable to carry out in Oslo were finally able to take place and resulted in another controversial deduction: cancerous tumors were a late-stage manifestation of a disease that has its roots in the sickness of society as whole, a sickness that prevented the proper expression and release of energy, causing stagnation or excesses which would result in malignancies or neuroses. The Orgone Accumulator could awaken the energy of those who had been suppressed into a state of dormancy, helping to regulate the energetic economy, but too much Orgone energy could engender problems of its own. Reich began to refine his research to address these issues and eventually The Function of the Orgasm and The Cancer Biopath would be translated re-published as Volumes I and II of The Discovery of Orgone, as he came to retrospectively understand the implications of his earlier work in light of his later discoveries.

Unfortunately, Reich was extremely misunderstood by his fellow scientists and society at large. He had immigrated to America with some political ideas that were unwelcome in the era of McCarthyism and so became a "person of interest" to Homeland Security officials, although by that stage of his life he was far less interested in promoting the Marxist political ideas that had made won him little favor in Europe, than he was in continuing his research in peace. It was concluded, however, that the mildly eccentric scientist was not a threat to national security as he spent most his time peering up at the sky on the rural ranch where his laboratory was based. For a while he was simply left alone with his "Orgone boxes" to establish the nature and properties of the energy that he saw everywhere and in everything.

In spite of the lack of support from the mainstream science community, Reich was not deterred from his study of the Orgone until a vicious newspaper article was published that heralded him as the leader of "The New Cult of Sex and Anarchy." This was a blatant and perhaps deliberate misinterpretation of Reich's idea that sexual energy and life energy were one and the same thing, and that healthy sexual expression was important to the overall health of the individual as well as society as a whole. This article brought Reich to the attention of the FDA, which then began to investigate him, apparently based on the suspicion that he was running some kind of perverted operation, using his scientific activities as a cover. Part of the misunderstanding could have been due to his infant research program, in which Reich naively sought to demonstrate how character armoring starts to present early on in children's development. Objections that were no doubt Puritanical in nature were raised, which led to the end of that particular program and so Reich returned to his environmental efforts where the nature of the aspersions that could be cast against him would not be quite so damning.

By the 1950s, Reich was seeing more than Orgone when he gazed out at the cosmos. His interest in the relationship between Orgone and atmospheric conditions had developed after his discovery of DOR from the ORANUR Experiments and led to the invention of the

Cloudbuster, with which he had hoped to draw off the deadened energy that persisted in the form of dense, unmoving black clouds. From observations of the sun and moon, fog and smoke, arid and rainy areas, Reich started to draw conclusions about the atmospheric interactions of Orgone, drawing parallels to the concepts of expansion and contraction of energy that he had observed in the bio-energy of the human body and even in bions themselves. In a series of "rain-making" experiments, Reich alleged that he could control the weather using his fantastical device.

Contracted OR	Expanded OR
Tendency toward:	Tendency toward:
Matter	Energy
Immobilization	Mobility
"cold", freezing	"heat" expansion
autumn, winter	spring, summer
strong potential differences	even distribution of OR energy

From The Orgone Institute, Vol VI, Nos 1-4, July 1954

The hours spent speculating on the sky ultimately resulted in some rather incredible observations, namely UFOs. Attested to by Reich and several of his assistants, strange objects began to appear in the sky during the "cosmic engineering" efforts with the Cloudbuster. Reich insists that he had even entered into battle with them on some occasions, pointing the Cloudbuster at the foreign vessels as if they were a stubborn patch of DOR. Apparently these spacecraft were indeed responsible for such an excess of DOR, which was in turn responsible for the increasing desertification of the planet and sickness of its inhabitants.

Just when Reich started to reach what some would definitely describe as the peak of madness, the FDA made their move. Whether it was to do with the suspicions of inappropriate sexual conduct or his extra-terrestrial exploits, it became clear that the agency was not happy with the research that was taking place at Orgonon and so they tried to take him to court based on the claim that he was fraudulently promoting medical cures, although he had never claimed to cure anything and was only interested in testing the potential of using such devices as an Orgone Accumulator in that way.

Reich declared that it was not for a judge to decide whether or not his scientific pursuits were valid and so refused to appear in court to defend his assertions about this vital life energy. This moment of misplaced hubris led to a federal injunction that banned the sale and interstate transport of the Orgone Accumulator and any promotional material. Unfortunately in the translation and republishing of his earlier books, *The Function of the Orgasm* and *The Cancer Biopathy*, Reich had re-branded them as Volume I and II of *The Discovery of Orgone* and updated them to include details on how the information in those books influenced his later discoveries. In spite of the fact that neither of these books made any of the claims that FDA said Reich was being investigated for, the FDA declared that they were supplementary literature that promoted the use of an Orgone Accumulator in healing cancer and other illnesses. Six tonnes of books and pamphlets were burned in New York in what has been described as a "blatant example of anti-Constitutional activity."

While Reich and his colleague, Dr Silvert, were held in federal prison, Reich continued to speculate on his theories, paying particular attention to what he believed was happening on a cosmic level. Some of his final conversations with his son are recorded in Peter Reich's haunting and whimsical memoir, Book of Dreams, in which he describes his experiences growing up at Orgonon. The memoir tells the story of the men in black cars who would come and interrogate Reich and the other scientists, up until the day they came and ordered the destruction of every Orgone Accumulator on the premises, a defeat which broke his heart. Peter recalls his father's insistence that he was targeted for his greater knowledge, that he would be dead before he could complete his work.

While in prison, Reich believed he had worked out the missing piece, the last bit of irrefutable evidence he needed to show that Orgone was not just a product of his imagination. He urged his son to be ready, for on his next visit he would need to pass this vital information on to him, to pass on to what was left of the team he had worked with before. There was no next visit. Wilhelm Reich's heart gave out before he could see his son again and the last piece of the Orgone puzzle died with him. In spite of all the good he intended to do for the world, the world had no such intention for him and so his legacy lives on, clouded by rumor and conspiracy, hidden truths and unproven claims.

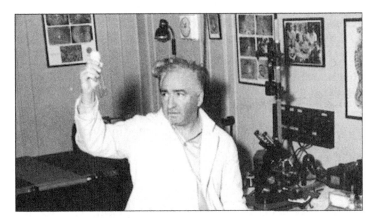

Wilhelm Reich in his Laboratory

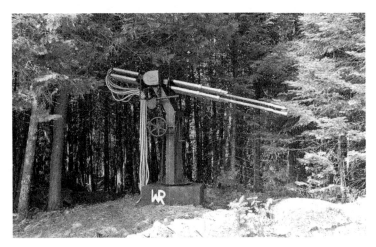

Original Cloudbuster

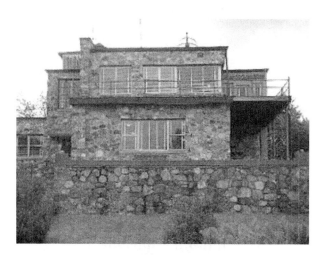

Orgonon

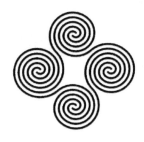

CHAPTER TWELVE

CULT AND CONSPIRACY

"The issue is clear: be destroyed or be proven correct. There is no other alternative."
•Wilhelm Reich [American Odyssey]

I n spite of his promising start in the field of psychoanalysis, Reich would ultimately be rejected by the group because of his Jewish heritage and alignment with Marxist politics. Whether out of self-preservation or simple disagreement, the Vienna Psychoanalytic Society expelled him from their ranks when the Nazi party started gaining political momentum in the early 1930s. The KPD (Communist party of Germany) of which Reich was a member was banned the day after Hitler came into power, and so Reich was forced to flee the country for his own safety. Because his books spoke of sexual liberation and freedom from fascist authoritarianism, it is no surprise that they were burned and banned in the city of Berlin where he had been carrying out his research and practice.

His interest in the underlying sexual nature of life in its entirety earned him little respect in Norway either where he was publicly vilified in a newspaper campaign denouncing him in part, due to his work which involved recording the bioelectric energy of humans in a state of sexual excitation. The main concern about this experiment was that some of the participants were not married. More importantly, he was denied access to funding because of his peers refusal to give his work a fair critique. In the words of his son, Peter Reich:

"His work was never disproven, only dismissed."

After being ousted from Scandinavia, Reich sought refuge from the second world war in the United States, where he was first investigated in the spirit of McCarthyism and later bore the misfortune of figure heading Mildred Bradie's smear campaign against psychoanalysis in general. The FDA banned his inventions and literature and imprisoned him. But these all happened in his lifetime and you've read about them in the biographical section already. This section is about the conspiracy that continues against him today, many years after his demise.

The first thing you will notice when reading through the results of an online search is the number of times the words "pseudoscience" or "fringe scientist" appear. There are references to Einstein, who had been interested in Reich's ORAC before dismissing the phenomena they observed as a simple convection effect a few weeks later. Of course, one is meant to read this and scoff that if a man as smart as Einstein didn't believe him, why should anyone else? But Einstein scoffed at the probability models of quantum mechanics too and that hasn't stopped an entire field of study from emerging. Of course, there are many entries for Reich and Orgone on a number of skeptics' blogs and websites, yet nearly all of them fail to conceal that they have done only the most rudimentary reading of his work, if any at all. What is the most striking is the sheer arrogance with which many of his detractors castigate him, without even realizing that they are "debunking" claims which were never made by Reich or any of his associates.

Critics will spend as much time coming up with reasons Reich couldn't possibly have discovered what he claims as it would take to simply try one of his experiments, without so much as looking at an Orgone Accumulator. A favorite is the problem of the microscope: Reich's notes record him looking at his samples at magnifications much greater than equipment at the time was able to clearly resolve, which is enough for many people to immediately cry out "Fraud!" and move on. If they had bothered to do further research, they would have learned that

Reich acknowledged that the lack of resolution made it impossible to observe details, but he was still able to see patterns of movement that indicated changes taking place in a supposedly dead and sterile solution, patterns that were inconsistent with regular Brownian motion.

To take it one step further, one could even investigate the Rife microscope, an instrument rumored to have been invented in the 1930s that has been all but erased from the history of science, which it is supposed Reich could have had access to. Rife's microscope was capable of much higher magnification than normal optical microscopes and had the advantage of being able to view living matter, something that an electron microscope cannot offer. What Rife could observe in minute detail was the behavior of cells as small as a virus and identify their unique resonance by tuning the frequency generator paired with his complex optical device. Rife believed he had discovered a microbial cause for cancerous tumors plague the human body and like any other scientist who has made this observation, suffered the fate of persecution and derision from orthodox microbiologists who have built their careers on observations of dead matter. Rife's frequencies are still used in sound and energetic healing in a similar to way to Radionics devices, although practitioners have to use clever wording to escape retribution from the AMA.

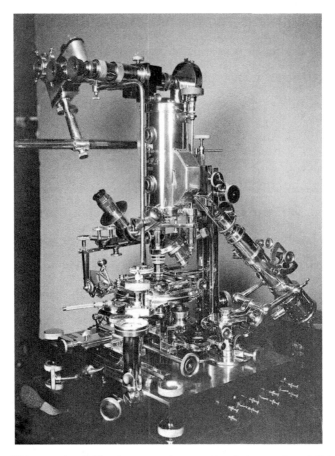

The incredibly complex Rife microscope that permitted observation of living viruses through light and resonance

More bizarre are the claims that Reich was fostering a culture of abuse, based on the actions of Albert Duvall and Felicia Saxe, who had studied his therapeutic techniques. The allegations of abuse of children by Reichian therapists is mostly found in conjunction with articles attempting to discredit Reich's work in its entirety by drawing attention to its most unorthodox elements and implying that Reich should somehow take responsibility for the actions of manipulative and abusive people that had shown an interest in his research or trained in Vegetotherapy. This appropriation of real people's traumatic experience is a discredit to both the victims and Dr Reich. His belief that early intervention in children could prevent the development of neurotic conditions in adulthood led him to begin a program of infant research, which he was forced to shut down after it was revealed that unscrupulous characters were taking advantage of children in their private practices. In hindsight, Reich's naiveté is obvious, but the fact remains that he was never accused of any misconduct and the attempts to conflate the actions of others with the man himself comes across as particularly disingenuous.

The authenticity of further attempts to discredit him are questionable due to the nature in which they are found; there are recurring comments across multiple platforms, particularly blog articles on Wilhelm Reich or book reviews. These boldly claim that Reich was a charlatan and abuser, yet further investigation yielded no sources other than a link back to the comment authors' own websites. Unsurprisingly, one of them was advertising a book in which they describe their personal traumatic childhood experience in the Orgone Accumulator, but only as a side note in an autobiographical novel that is primarily about pursuing an intimate relationship with a dolphin. The other commentator who was found on several pages is a software engineer with a science-fiction webpage, with a section dedicated entirely to debunking Reich and all of his work. His umbrage seems to come as a result of childhood victimization by the same Albert Duvall recounted by other unfortunate individuals. The rest of his website includes a number of parody articles and stories. It's all rather odd and I encourage the reader to do their own investigations, if not to understand more about Reich's theory of Orgone, then at least to see the open display of contempt for a man who simply wanted make people, society and the planet itself healthier.

One of the most outrageous posthumous allegations against Reich comes from Al Bielek, by way of Don Croft and invokes the infamous Montauk Project. For those unfamiliar with this classic conspiracy theory, it features all the usual hallmarks: Shady CIA operatives, secret underground bases, time travel, mind control and heinous treatment of young men and boys. As a supposed survivor of the project, Al recounts that Wilhelm Reich was among the first scientists to work at the facility, sought out for his knowledge regarding the power of sexual energy and its influence on psychology. The story continues with Reich refusing to participate after learning the true nature of the experiments that took place at this secret government site, but there is no evidence that places him there, or anyone else. Don Croft first reported hearing this story from Bielek directly, in his logs of a cross-country gifting excursion, although it was also mentioned in several lectures and videos from the 1990s. In the 1992 book The Montauk Project, author Preston B Nicholls suggests that Reich was first recruited for his weather engineering efforts and only later approached to consult on the matter of bioelectricity and biological programming. It seems that there is no known source placing Reich there, although a memo from

MKULTRA from 1960 alludes to the potential study of bioelectricity as a means for remote control of the human organism, although it is dated 1960, three years after Reich's death. Several articles allude to the FBI folder on Reich; however, the links are no longer active, nor does the file seem to be available on the vault. Several requests for information have been made under the FOIA, sometimes repeatedly, but it seems the traces of Reich are disappearing from public view once again.

Currently the study of Orgonomy lives on through several small institutions in the United States and around the world. Orgonomists are limited in the work that they are able to carry out due to the dangers of working with Oranur and DOR, so there is a stronger emphasis on the biological and therapeutic areas of study. Recently, in a book publish by Harvard Edu, James Strick, co-director of the Reich Trust re-examines the Bion experiments and suggests it's time that the world takes a closer look at what Reich discovered all those years ago. Strick gives a concise analysis of the way Rockefeller funding diverted the path of science to suit the reductionist agenda of the time and what that meant for those who were not prepared to simply adjust to the new status quo. Reich is the prime example of a scientist that found himself in such a position and it is worth perusing Strick's articles and videos to see it all in context.

Reich's psychoanalytical theories fared far better than his cosmic theories. They were hardly taken seriously until the 1970s, when a student of Geography and Climate Science by the name of James DeMeo applied for permission to research the more unorthodox parts of Reich's legacy. DeMeo had always been interested in the concept of the ether, in particular he was fascinated by the famous null result of the Michelson-Morley experiment and couldn't understand why the physics community interpreted the results the way they did. Still today there are more-than-qualified physicists who think that the world was too hasty to dismiss the possible existence of an etheric field, simply because a static ether had been disproven.

James DeMeo went on to become a professor of Earth, Atmospheric and Environmental Sciences and continued to investigate Reich's theories, particularly in relation to desert climates. He undertook his own climate engineering projects using the Cloudbuster, the results of which he has published in various studies and books. He is still actively researching Orgone at his lab in Oregon. DeMeo has established himself as an independent authority on all things Orgone…except orgonite that is. Along with the institutions that continue Reich's original work, he unequivocally denounces "the current craze about 'orgonite', 'orgonium', 'orgone generators', 'orgone zappers', 'chembusters' and similar distortions" as a rationality-breaching misrepresentation of Reich's ideas. Although no studies have been done, it seems that there is very little interest in the idea of an orgone-matrix material from the Orgonomy community.

The ideas that Reich left behind were handed over to a trust that he formed before his death, which he had hoped his daughter, Dr Eva Reich would take on. She was not in a position to do so at the time of his death, neither were there any willing ex-colleagues or students to be found. Thus, the responsibility eventually fell on the shoulders of a patient who had had much success with Reichian therapy and felt compelled to maintain the museum at Orgonon in spite of the insufficient funding available in the trust. Mary Boyd Higgins ran the trust until her passing in 2019, which was heralded in a blog entry by one Joel Carlinsky under the heading "Ding dong, the witch is dead" which of course led down another alleyway of intrigue. Carlinsky, at one time a student of Eva Reich, maintains that Boyd-Higgins was complicit in preventing access to Reich's original documents, which prevented scholars from understanding the true scope of his work and allowed his reputation to be further tarnished by the continued misinterpretation of his efforts.

Carlinsky runs a blog titled "Deconstructing Orgonomy" in which he points out all of the flaws, misappropriation of ideas, and corruption that he believes is happening in the community, in an effort to return to the essence of the subject itself. In 2014 he wrote:

"As long as it is impossible to bring up bions or cloudbusting in a conversation with a scientist without getting bogged down in pointless digressions about UFOs, Communist plots, military secrets, sex, right-wing political ideologies, psychotherapy and the personality of a man who has now been dead for two generations, there will never be any serious discussion of orgonomic scientific findings. The life and personality of Reich…still overshadows everything he touched."

This seems like a rational statement to make, although James DeMeo and several others report that Carlinsky is a public menace that has made it his business to denounce Wilhelm Reich's work as well as those who continue it. There are reports that he has harassed people in their homes and broken into the Reich Museum to get his hands on original materials, flown long-distance to interfere with ongoing research investigations and many more distressing incidents. Between DeMeo and Carlinsky is a history of contention to rival that of Karl Welz and Don Croft. Unfortunately, it is no more apparent who is in the right than who was the first to truly invent orgonite, as both men have been duly discredited by at least one educational institution, a badge of honor worn proudly by all of those who skirt the edges and push the boundaries of established thought.

The more you look around, the more it becomes clear that the impression that the so-called reputable institutions want you to have of Reich is that he was a nut, a man who would have been better off writing science fiction than actually doing science. But many others believe that in the case of Reich, the establishment does indeed protest too much. In an emerging power structure that was more fragile than it seemed, his open-minded and multidisciplinary approach was perceived as a threat because it exposed the inner workings of a system that can only work if the people are blind to the mechanism. This dynamic between Reich as an individual and the establishments of socio-politics and science were explored best in a documentary called

Who's Afraid of Wilhelm Reich? which is a great place to start diving deeper into this fascinating story. Another documentary that highlights the pointed rejection of Reich's theories is Man's Right to Know. Although Reich may seem somehow quaint or comical from our perspective, it is important to remember that we are in a unique position in terms of our relationship with people and institutions of power. There is far more transparency and individual autonomy now than was even possible, never mind permissible in Reich's time. He flew dangerously close to the sun with his keen and accurate criticisms of power structures and even closer still to what many believe are far more sacred truths about the nature of reality. Unfortunately, his earnest and slightly unsophisticated demeanour made it too easy to discredit him and ultimately make a fool of him so that his work would be dismissed as the idle ramblings of a sex-obsessed, UFO-spotting wannabe scientist.

The truth often depends entirely on what you believe in. Many people already reject the idea of an etheric energy and so there is no point in going any further. Others are happy to explore the idea of a life force energy that can be tapped into, but draw the line at aliens. If you are on board with aliens, then inter-dimensional cosmic warfare isn't such a reach.

With Reich and Orgone, it's a matter of where you choose to draw the line, and in terms of orgonite, it's pretty clear where the divide lies. Karl Welz hardly references Reich's cosmic theories, only the concept of Orgone itself and its polar twin, DOR. Don Croft, on the other hand, tirelessly dedicated decades of his life to dismantling the cosmic corruption caused by extradimensional entities using frequency-charged crystals embedded in an orgone matrix.

The question is never was there a conspiracy against Reich, but rather why he was conspired against. The plainest answer is that he simply hit the nail too squarely on the head with his critique of governments and the organization of society. Perhaps it was in their best interest that his ideas did not get the opportunity to enter the domain of popular thought. It could be because there is a well-funded pathway that steers scientists away from investigating the innate electricity of the human body and the environment, diverting research away from holistic and non-medical therapies that don't require repeat prescriptions or can't be sold at a profit. Lastly the conspiracy could be that all these things are true because Reich really did uncover the underlying fabric of the universe to make contact with space and came far too close to exposing that everything, we know is just an illusion in a much, much more terrifying reality.

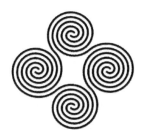

CHAPTER THIRTEEN

THE YOGA OF ORGONE

C haos. Order. Entropy. Growth. Yin and Yang, Shiva and Shakti. We live in a world of dualities and polarities, similarities and opposites, parallels and perpendiculars. We also live in a world of tangents and spirals and something that is so elusive to our science that it might as well be called magic and that is life. Spiritualists will talk of the Razor's Edge, the narrow path where worlds intersect, where all is one and the opposites and parallels are revealed to be the illusions that they truly are. Reich and the students that came after him may not have believed in this path in the same way, but they understood that they were working with a force so pervasive as to be barely measurable and the effects were obvious to anyone who took the time to see for themselves.

Reich's understanding of orgastic potential resonates with many people who are familiar with the concept of kundalini, which comes from the ancient philosophies of tantra. Although Reich insisted that his treatments were not yoga, even going so far as to say "this is not yoga" when guiding a patient through a breathing technique, I am inclined to believe his impression of yoga might have been somewhat superficial, given the era. The strange art of traveling swamis had not yet evolved into a popular activity in Europe or America in the early 20th Century and even in India it was practiced in a very ascetic and celibate way under the influence of religious colonization. We are currently at a point in time where many nations enjoy the freedom to explore their own history and culture as well as others and have the privilege of advanced education and technology with which to do so. As a result we know much more now about the confluence of "eastern" and "western" traditions than Reich would have.

Even with this in mind, it seems slightly incredible that he would fail to see the similarities between the Vedic concept of prana and his own Orgone. Perhaps if the prudish Europeans weren't so intent on prohibiting discussion on sexual matters, he might have come across a description of the Kundalini Tantra and unlocked a new dimension to his work. As it was, he was already treated like a deviant for daring to write about sex at all, so it is perhaps unlikely that this discovery would have done him any favors in terms of public perception. The famous guru Rajneesh, also known as Osho, recognized Reich as a Tantric master for his work with energy and empathized with his rejection from the polite society of his time. Osho further expressed his support of Reich's ideas by installing a large Orgone Accumulator known as The Egg at his ashram in Pune to facilitate deeper meditations among the gurukul. Like the Tantrics, Reich had understood the implicit magic of sexual energy and begun to explore the relationship of the charge and discharge of orgastic potential with the equilibrium of the psyche. One of the main esoteric practices in regard to sexual energy is that of transmutation. The sexual energy is considered the most powerful, in part because it is so tangibly embodied. With certain techniques, tantrics and kundalini practitioners can expand or contract energy from the sexual center and move it perceptibly through the body with the idea of ascending to higher frequency and heightened consciousness.

The Hatha Yoga Pradipika expresses the importance of purifying the channels through which prana, or energy, travels before undertaking any breathing exercises designed to influence or amplify the prana in your body. It is stated very clearly that a failure to do so will exacerbate any existing negative conditions afflicting the mind or body of the practitioner. This is very similar to what Reich discovered with his Orgone devices: the energy does not discern; it simply goes where it has access to. Stepping into an Orgone Accumulator or practicing yoga doesn't increase the amount of energy, it simply increases how much of it becomes accessible to you, or rather, how much of you becomes accessible to it. Like Reich putting radioactive substances in the accumulator, opening up your body to free range life force energy is just not a good idea until you know what you're doing.

In Christian communities, awakening the Kundalini is considered to be dark magic of the highest order. Online you can find pages and pages of testimonials describing the dangers and ill effects of awakening the serpent energy. This seems fair enough, considering that in Christian lore, the snake that leads Eve to the tree of knowledge is ultimately to blame for the corruption of human innocence. Although practitioners of yoga may consider the reasoning behind this apprehension misguided, it is not entirely misplaced. The dangers of experiencing a spontaneous Kundalini awakening are touted as much by yogis as they are by evangelicals, as it can often bear all the hallmarks of a nervous breakdown. One does not simply tap into a raw electrical current without making sure they have a closed and complete circuit, with the right transformers and conducting materials in place.

To do this with yoga, you need to practice a series of breathing techniques and postures that break up tension or blockages in the body and you need to meditate, allowing the brainwaves to enter a relaxed state which facilitates healing in the body by activating the parasympathetic nervous system. Once you have optimized the energetic ecosystem of your own mind and body, you can advance to the techniques that amplify or increase the flow of prana. In Reichian therapy, you would dissolve the "armouring" of the body and character with a series of breathing techniques and physical manipulations by the therapist, which act upon the vegetative system, which is the name previously used to describe the parasympathetic nervous system.

There is yet another similarity between Hatha Yoga and Vegetotherapy: the seven rings. Hatha yoga uses a seven-chakra system that situates vortices of energy along the spine, from the pelvis to the crown of the head. Each chakra governs a specific set of functions in the body and mind as well as helping to manage the subtle energy flow. Exhibitions of strength or weakness can be attributed to "open" or "blocked" chakras, which means the vortex of energy is not moving to project energy in the way it should be and the result manifests as a physical or mental dysfunction.

In Vegetotherapy, therapists work according to seven distinct segments of the body that display unique characteristics of muscular armoring as a result of emotional or energetic tension. Hardening of the musculature in a particular segment represents a stagnation of energy in the system that can perpetuate physical or psychic illness. These segments are also mapped along the spine, from pelvis to head and although there are minor differences in placement when compared with chakras, the result is the same. Both systems are geared towards creating and maintaining a healthy and optimized flow of energy in the body. According to Reich, conscious liberation can only be reached when the armoring of the body and mind has been dissolved. Likewise in yoga, liberation of the self requires the ascension of the kundalini through open and unblocked chakras.

Several experiments have been done to try and find scientific proof of chakras, using techniques similar to Reich's original research into bio-electricity. Both parapsychologist and philosopher Dr Hiroshi Matoyama and kinesiologist and UCLA researcher Valerie Hunt have performed extensive electrode-based experiments that measure distinct changes in energy readings from the body when chakras are activated through meditative or physical processes. These experiments imply that the human body is equipped with psycho-physical links between matter and pure energy.

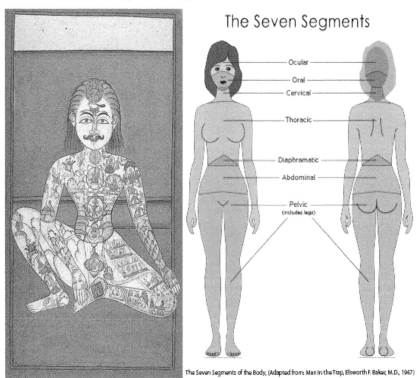

The Seven Segments

Ocular
Oral
Cervical
Thoracic
Diaphramatic
Abdominal
Pelvic
(includes legs)

The Seven Segments of the Body, (Adapted from: Man in the Trap, Elsworth F. Baker, M.D., 1967)

The 7 main chakras of Hatha Yoga

What makes this all interesting in regard to orgonite is that our bones themselves are a composite matrix of organic and inorganic matter, which means that every bone in the body could potentially be acting in the same way as an orgone matrix. Even the connective tissues are formed as a matrix of living cells and inorganic ground substance, which means the spine is made up of layers of differently composed matrices. As it is the foundation for our major electrical infrastructure, namely the nerves, the spine is of unique importance in the electric body, even without application of esoteric thought. It provides the framework for a system which carries a great deal of information that allows us to interact with the material universe by transmitting and receiving electrical impulses from the brain.

In yoga, it is believed that the most important energy channel of the body, shushumna, travels right through the center of the spine. Ascension of energy through this channel is one of the key aims of yoga. Practices in yoga and vegetotherapy aim to engage the autonomic nervous system in a controlled manner that helps to improve the neural network of the brain and body as a whole, which means enhancing the distribution of energy. In the previous chapters, we discussed how Orgone energy can be restructured when an electrical charge is applied to a matrix of organic and inorganic materials, so the body in this context could be viewed as a system that can effectively generate and restructure primordial energy. There are a number of techniques that greatly enhance its ability to do so.

In an interview with renowned breatharian, Elitom Elohim, we spoke about his experience with orgonite. Elitom teaches the advanced spiritual practice of subsisting solely off of etheric energy, that is living without eating. He recognizes that Orgone is simply another word for prana, qi or mana and orgonite is simply a tool that teaches us about the true nature of energy and how to access it.

"All these words deal with the same thing," he laughs. *"They just come from different cultures. Reich got the word orgone, from orgasm, because he understood that in nature, everything is always reproducing itself and therefore the nature of the fundamental energy is innately sexual. Even the cells of our body reproduce as the energy flows. He used the word orgone to refer to the earth and the atmosphere - all of it - and taught people how to use natural materials to set things up within that to grab the energy flow from the atmosphere to use freely."*

Elitom talks about the human body as the "first wireless technology", not only bringing up a reference to the spine as the battery of the body but also pointing out the importance of grounding the body by walking barefoot, allowing electrons to pass up the body and charge it up. For Elitom, who slept on an orgone-accumulating pillow made of layers of steel wool and cotton in the early days of his practice, the process of learning how to make orgonite led him to a much greater understanding about how much energy is available and how easy it is to gain access to it once you become aware of how it is attracted and repelled.

"And it's really fun!" he adds, pointing out that anything that feels good to do and teaches you something at the same time is a worthwhile endeavor.

"Free energy is all around us and we should know how to tap into it. Free energy is breathwork, feng shui, having fun, being creative and imparting the most positive energy. We are the only animal that has the power to completely transform our external environment. You can use that power to bring more energy into your spaces and change the entire atmosphere. You can charge your food, your water, your pillow...I have a friend who is building a floor out of orgonite in his house! The more materials you use and the bigger it is, the more energy you get."

AFTERWORD

THE FUTURE OF ORGONITE

Looking to the future, orgonite is not going away any time soon. In fact, it seems to be becoming more popular, with more and more people learning how to make it themselves.

Even within the mainstream science of nanotechnology, polymer matrix materials are being explored for the suspension and stabilization of metallic nanoparticles in microgels for high end technological applications including photonics - the branch of science that studies the properties of photons and especially their potential application as a medium for transmitting information.

Although some of the alternative modes of science discussed in this book are consistently derided by the current scientific establishment, so to speak, there is no shortage of intelligent, credentialled people and organisations who are open-minded and willing to explore the potentials offered by these models. Even if they lack empirical proof of effects, they offer perspectives that can influence the approach of more accepted and established processes.

Orgonite represents a step away from the confines of politically controlled science; an exploration into alternative ways of interacting with energy, radiation, matter and information. It demonstrates what it means to approach science holistically, moving beyond reductionism and accepting that there are unseen forces which shape our pathways through reality. When we question something as simple as orgonite, we are invited to question things that we would otherwise blindly accept and it encourages us to know more about the world around us.

BIBLIOGRAPHY & REFERENCES

Chapter 1:

Difference Between Orgonium And Orgonite – Orgonite Crystal Orgone Articles – Orgone Energy Australia Who Was Dr. Wilhelm Reich? And Why Has History Tried So Hard To Erase Him?

Chapter 2:

Orgone Energy Reich and Welz Karl Welz – Orgone Generator orgone generators, orgonite and stale orgone energy (DOR) The Complete Guide to Orgone Generators (2019) | Orgone Generator® Orgone Adventures for www.educate-yourself.org Orgonite & Tactical Orgone Gifting | View Forum - Questions and Answers Orgonite PDFs – Etheric Warriors – Undermining tyranny with simple orgonite FW: And - does orgonite really work? - Check The Evidence

Chapter 3:

C.O.R.E (Cosmic Orgone Engineering), Wilhelm Reich M.D., Publications of the Orgone Institute, Vol. VI, Nos. 14 [July 1954] On Wilhelm Reich and Orgonomy, James DeMeo [1993] Bion-Biogenesis Research and Seminars at OBRL: Progress Report. Pulse of the Planet. 5. 100-113., James DeMeo [2002] Experimental Confirmation of the Reich Orgone Accumulator Thermal Anomaly, James DeMeo Subtle Energies & Energy Medicine • Volume 20 • Number 3 What is Orgone Energy?, Charles R Kelley [1962 Bioenergy and Orgone Matrix Material: A Primer, John Logan [2005] Org]one Biophysics | The Institute for Orgonomic Science Orgone Energy Neutralizes Nuclear Radiation: The ORANUR Experiment Reich's Radiation Disaster - Stillness in the Storm James DeMeo's Research Website - On Wilhelm Reich & Orgone Energy Experiments regarding the existence of orgone | Hellenic Institute of Orgonomy The orgone accumulator's effectiveness as evidenced by the Reich Blood Test – YouTube

Chapter 4:

Adventures in the Orgasmatron: How the Sexual Revolution Came to America, Christopher Turner [2011] ORGONE ENERGY | the-chembow Orgone Energy | Georg Ritschl – YouTube

Chapter 5:

An Introduction to Orgonite Matrix Material, Jon Logan [2004] The Healing Universe. Scalar Energy and Healing | Life Energy Designs Orgonite Inventor - How to Make Orgonite - YouTube Orgonite & Tactical Orgone Gifting | View topic - Kirlian Photos of different types of orgonite.

Chapter 6:

Picture of water in cloud buster pipes. ICE TEST - ORGONE PYRAMID PART 2 - YouTube Orgonite & gardening/farming The Orgonite Experiment. How to super-size your vegetables Orgone and Lemon Experiment after 1 month Part 2 - YouTube Visible effect of orgone on the atmosphere

Chapter 7:

Framework for developing health-based EMF standards, World Health Organization [2006] Radiation Studies - CDC: Non-Ionizing RadiationNon-Ionizing Radiation - Overview | Occupational Safety and Health Administration Frequency List – Orgone Generator Extremely Low Frequency (ELF) Radiation - Health Effects | Occupational Safety and Health Administration

Chapter 8:

Casimir force: The Quantum Around You. Ep 6 - YouTube Piezoelectric Effect - an overview | ScienceDirect Topics

Chapter 9:

The Function of the Orgasm, Wilhelm Reich, M.D. The Cancer Biopathy, Wilhelm Reich, M.D. Experiment XX Wilhelm Reich, Orgone Energy and UFOs, Peter Robbins [2011] What Is Orgone Energy?, Charles R Kelley, Ph. D [1962] Book of Dreams, Peter Reich [1973] Turkish experiment

Chapter 10:

Einstein: "Ether and Relativity" - MacTutor History of Mathematics Atomic Geometry - In2infinity Hydrogen Wave Function 1 - Tales of the Dodecahedron

Chapter 11:

The Passion of Youth, Wilhelm Reich, M.D. The Function of the Orgasm, Wilhelm Reich, M.D. The Cancer Biopathy, Wilhelm Reich, M.D. Man of Fury, Myron Sharaf In Defense of Wilhelm Reich, James DeMeo United States v. the Wilhelm Reich Foundation, 17 F.R.D. 96 (D. Me. 1954) Wilhelm Reich Overview A Time Line – Wilhelm Reich and the Science of Life Energy | The Journal of Psychiatric Orgone Therapy Wilhelm Reich | Project Gutenberg Self-Publishing - eBooks | Read eBooks online The American College of Orgonomy Orgone.org | Dr. Reich Sexual Energy Research Gets A Second Look - CBS News The Wilhelm Reich Pardon Project

Chapter 12:

The Montauk Project: Experiments in Time, Preston B Nichols, Peter Moon [1992] Wilhelm Reich, Biologist, James Strick, Ph.D. [2015] Orgone: cosmic pulse of life | Science | The Guardian Wilhelm Reich, Biologist by James Strick, Ph.D. Deconstructing Orgonomy James Strick Bion Experiments - YouTube A Skeptical Scrutiny of the Works and Theories of Wilhelm Reich Wilhelm Reich : Orgone Motor The Dangerous Truth about Orgone | Mysterious Universe Wilhelm Reich | Field Work Archives of the Orgone Institute - Wilhelm Reich

Museum www.orgonecontinuum.org: The Orgone Motor Growing Nonsense About Reich and Orgone on Global Internet Response to Irrational Critics and So-Called "Skeptics" What has become of the Rife Microscope - Royal Rife Research - Europe Al Bielek - The History of Montauk Project - YouTube TOXIC DISINFORMATION - Joel Carlinsky

Chapter 13:

Character Analysis: Part III, Wilhelm Reich, M.D., Farrar, Straus & Giroux, New York [1972] Kundalini Tantra, Swami Satyananda Saraswati, Bihar School of Yoga [1984] Infinite Mind: Science of the Human Vibrations of Consciousness, Valerie V. Hunt, Malibu Pub [1996] Theories of the Chakras: Bridge to Higher Consciousness, Dr Hiroshi Motoyama, [1982]

Chapter 14:

Polymer-matrix stabilized metal nanoparticles: Synthesis, characterizations and insight into molecular interactions between metal ions, atoms and polymer moieties - ScienceDirect Orgonite World Wide | Leading Orgonite and Orgone Zapper manufacturer | Free world wide shipping available

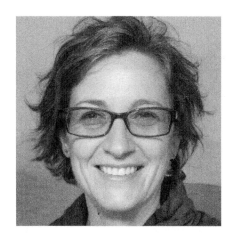

ABOUT THE AUTHOR

TERICA L. BRINK

Terica L. Brink is a first-time author and a full-time certified yoga instructor with a deep interest in the holistic wellness practices of the natural world. Drawing on her personal practice and research, Terica offers a comprehensive guide to the history, science, and practical applications of orgonite. As a yoga instructor, she is particularly interested in the ways in which orgonite can support physical, emotional, and spiritual well-being. With her clear and engaging writing style, Terica invites readers on a journey of discovery, and personal transformation, encouraging them to unlock the full potential of orgonite and the mysteries of the orgone matrix.

Printed in Great Britain
by Amazon